FITNESS SUTRA

Exercises with

Resistance Loop Bands

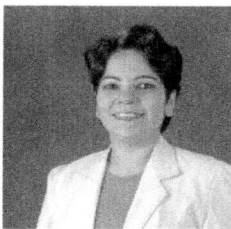

Dr. Monika Chopra
www.fitness-sutra.com

Although I am a Physiotherapist (PT, for those of you in the USA) and a trained Yoga teacher, my suggestions through this book do not establish a doctor-patient relationship between us. This book is not intended to be a substitute for the medical advice of physicians. You should regularly consult a physician in matters relating to your health particularly with respect to any symptoms that may require diagnosis or medical attention. I advise you to take full responsibility of your safety and be aware of your physical limits. Before practising the exercises described in this book, be sure that your equipment is well maintained. Do not take risks beyond your level of flexibility, aptitude, strength, and comfort level.

This is a work of nonfiction. No names have been changed, no characters invented and no events fabricated. The information provided within this Book is for general informational purposes only. While I have tried to keep the information up-to-date and correct, there are no representations or warranties, expressed or implied, about the completeness, accuracy, reliability, suitability or availability with respect to the information, products, services, or related graphics contained in this book for any purpose. Any use of this information is at the reader's own responsibility. I do not assume and hereby disclaim any liability to any party for any loss, damage, or disruption caused by errors or omissions, whether such errors or omissions result from negligence, accident, or any other cause.

CONTENTS

AN INTRODUCTION TO RESISTANCE LOOP BANDS

Resistance loop band training is a simple and effective way of doing your resistance exercise to increase muscle tone, muscle strength, burn fat or simply increase body flexibility. It is very cost effective and can be used on the go. It is safe for the beginners and at the same time can be made very challenging for intermediate and advance trainers.

In this book, through step by step instructions, I will guide you to the safe and effective methods of using resistance loop bands. Emphasis will be laid on the correct grasping of the band, proper start position and correct movement of the particular body part for the desired results.

Finally I will guide you to beginners, intermediate and advance training regimes which will help you to set desired goals.

What are resistance loop bands and how are they more useful than free weights or resistance bands?

Resistance loop bands are the resistance bands that come in the form of one continuous loop. With the loop you can perform the resistance exercises better than the conventional resistance band unit by targeting the workout of a specific muscle. One specific advantage of resistance loop band is that, as you stretch the loop band the resistance level increases thus providing a progressive increase in the muscle stress, which cannot occur with conventional free weights.

With resistance loop band you can do whole range of exercises involving all muscles of your body in various ways. These can also be used in conjunction with conventional exercises, thus making them more challenging or more achievable.

Why resistance loop bands?

Resistance loop bands have been used since ages for rehabilitation purpose. They provide a safe and effective method to strengthen up the muscles, ligaments, tendons and joints. Off late their popularity have increased amongst fitness enthusiasts because of ease and effectiveness of their usage. With just your body and your band you're not too far from the gym.

Here are some of the benefits of resistance loop training.

1. They are effective in strength training exercises.
2. They can be used anywhere- home, office and outdoors.
3. They are portable and storable. They take up little space and are lighter than the free weights.
4. They are extremely cost effective alternative to purchasing bulky gym equipment or taking expensive gym memberships.
5. Resistance loop bands are more versatile as they don't work against force of gravity. They are able to provide freer Range of motion than barbells or dumbbells.
6. With resistance loop bands muscles can work both through concentric and eccentric parts of an exercise.

Resistance loop band strength levels

Resistance loop bands have a restoring force that comes in action when the loop is stretched. This restoring force or resistance is linear in nature and varies with the stretch i.e. the more the band is stretched the more is the resistance force. This linear variable resistance helps to engage the fast twitch muscle fibre effectively, thus strengthening them better. Resistance loop band training when combined with free weights provide isotonic workout with linear resistance training which provides better body toning and strengthening.

The resistance level of most band systems follow a colour coded system based on the thickness of the band. The thicker the band, the more is the resistance level. You would need to refer to the band resistance chart of your loop bands.

While there are a number of resistance bands available in the market, I have found the Fitlastics range pretty good in quality. Their resistance levels and colour codes are given below for reference. If however you are using some other bands, then please refer to their respective colour coding.

Band Colour	Resistance Levels
Yellow	Extra Light
Green	Light
Red	Medium
Blue	Heavy
Black	Extra Heavy

RESISTANCE LOOP BAND BASICS

Grips

Up Grip

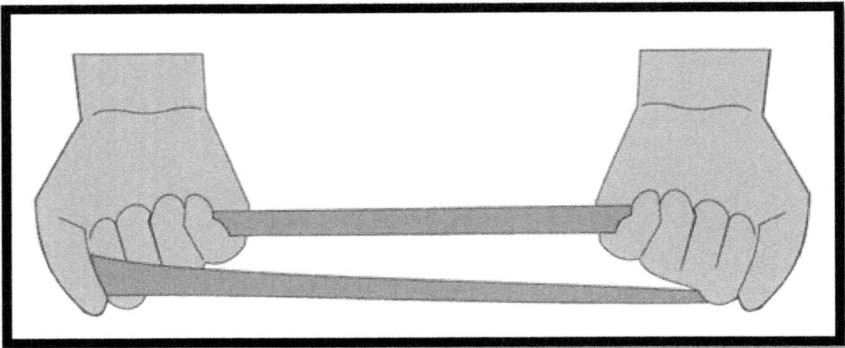

In up grip the band is held in the palms facing up, with fingers enclosing the band fully. It is mainly used in exercises where you have to curl or row the band towards your body, such as biceps curls.

Down Grip

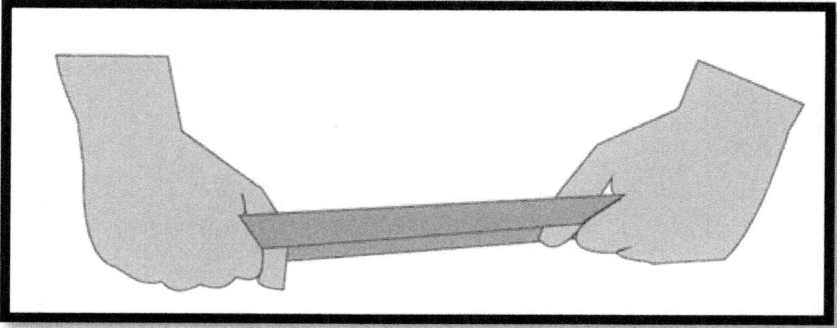

In down grip the band is held in the palms facing down, with fingers enclosing the band fully. It is mainly used for exercises which involve pushing the band away from your body (with the aid of a fixed anchor) or those that have you pulling the resistance toward you.

Hammer Grip

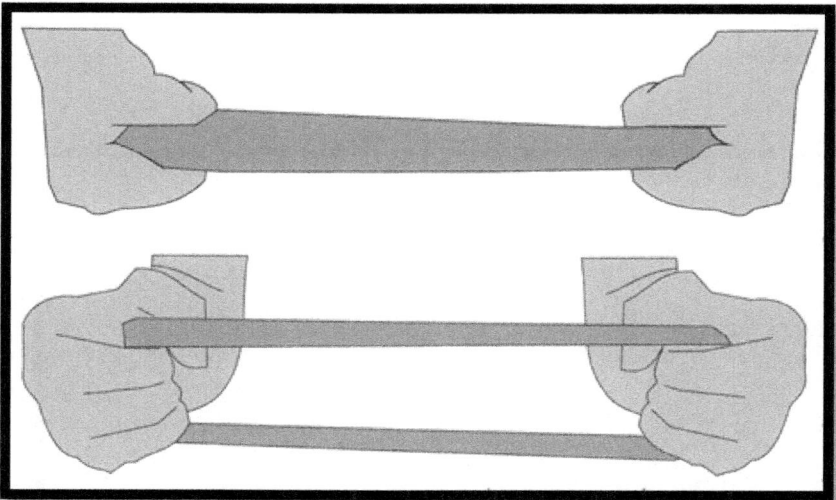

In hammer grip you hold the band in your fist, with both palms facing each other.

Open Hand Grip

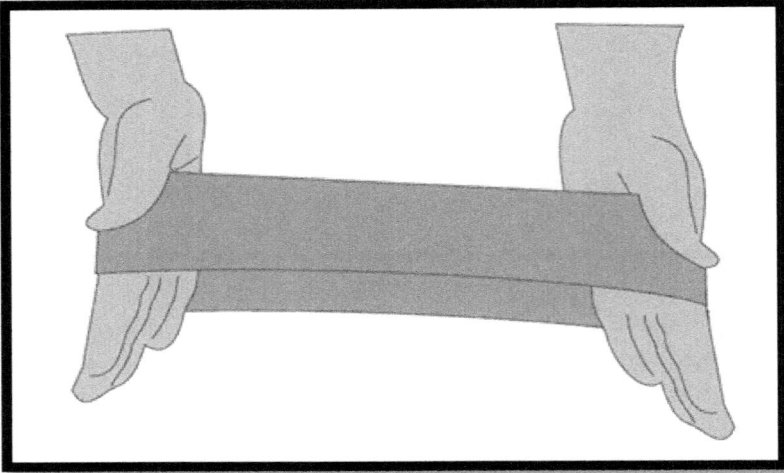

In open hand grip the band is wrapped around the open hands. It is normally used in pulling the band away from the body.

Wrist Alignment

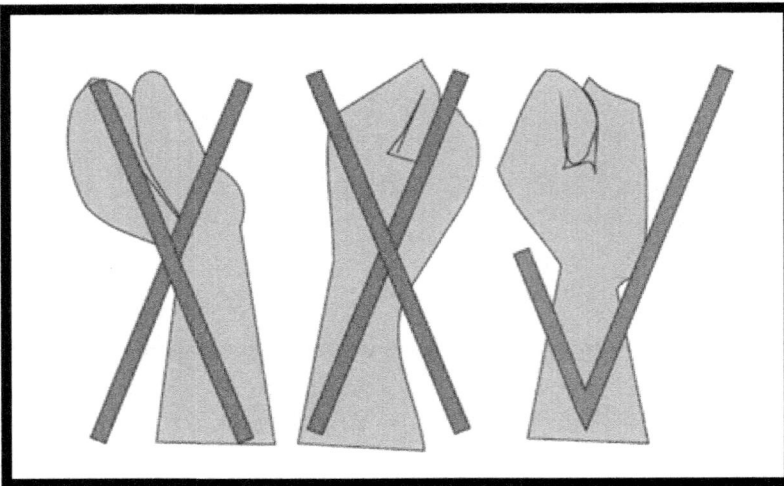

The band should be held in hand with wrist in neutral position i.e. hand should be in line with the forearm (neither extended nor flexed).

Ready Position

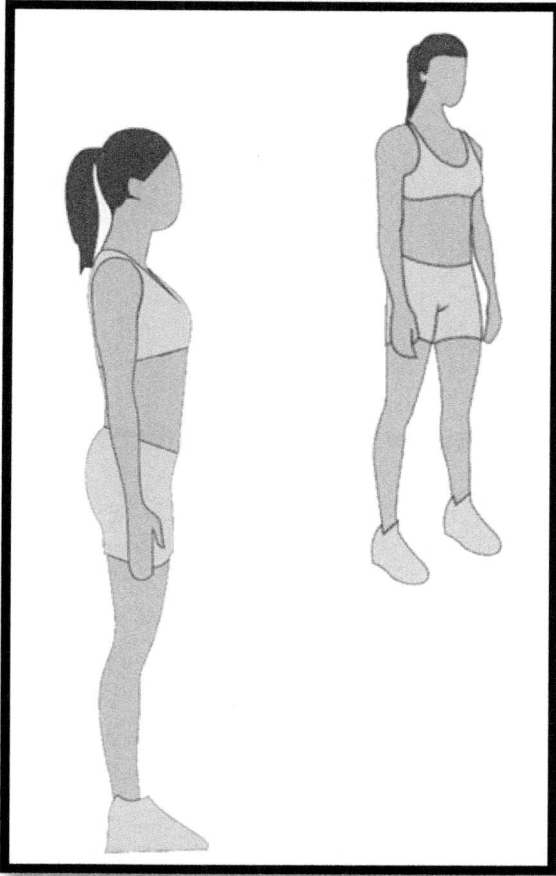

Stand tall with your feet hip width distance apart, shoulders and hips squared (facing forward), gluteal (hip) muscles contracted, knees soft with thigh muscles contracted, arms by the side of your body and looking straight forward

How to use the Band

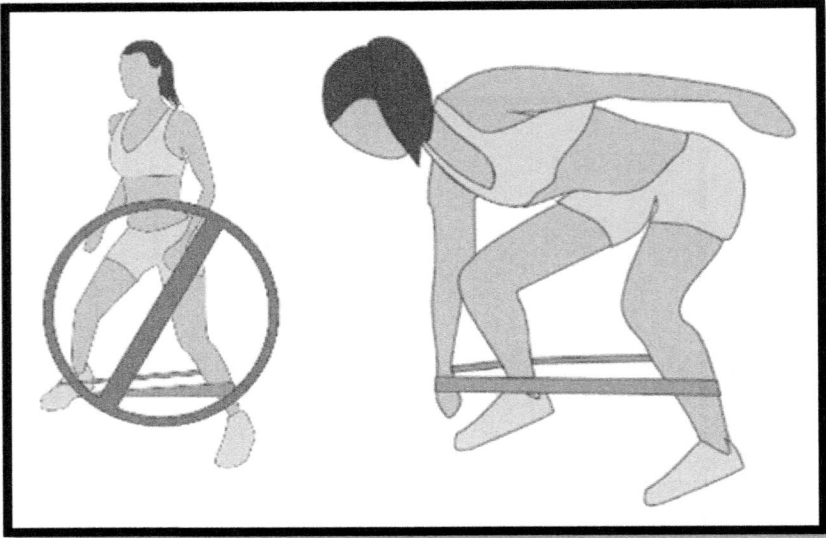

- Use the band only as directed.
- Never stretch the band towards face or other sensitive parts of the body.
- Never stretch the band more than 2½ times its resting length.
- If desired resistance is not achieved, when using according to directions, switch to a band that provides desired resistance.
- Inspect for possible wear and tear before use. Discontinue use if torn.
- Do not use on abrasive surface.
- Keep away from children.
- Perform your workout on carpeted surface, wood floors or grass. Abrasive surface like cement or asphalt can damage the band.

Make sure that when you put a resistance loop band around your ankles, you put it around your feet with both hands. When you take it off, make sure you take it off with both hands. Do not kick them off or try to take them off with your shoes. Doing so can damage the band.

WARM-UP EXERCISES

To stay safe and prepare your body for exercises you should always do some warm ups before the resistance exercises. The warm up exercises help to increase the temperature and loosen the muscles before the heavy body muscle work. Warm ups improve the body performance and prevent injuries. These exercises should be dynamic exercises like skipping, jogging at a place, chest expansion & rotations. About 5 minutes' warm ups are enough to make your cardiovascular system ready.

The following warm up exercises are good to prepare your body for intense workout (Do 10 repetitions per exercise)

1.   <u>Neck Rotations:</u>

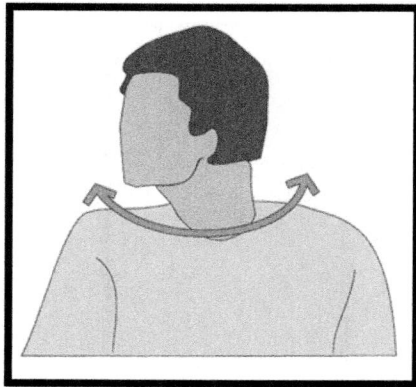

Stand tall with your chin parallel to the ground. Exhale and take your chin to the chest. Inhale, rotate your neck and take your chin towards the left shoulder (look over your left shoulder). Exhale and get your chin back to the chest position. Inhale, rotate your neck and take your chin to the right shoulder (look over your right shoulder). Get your chin back to the chest position as you exhale. Move you chin up to the start position as you inhale. Repeat 3 times.

2.   Shoulder Backward Rotations:

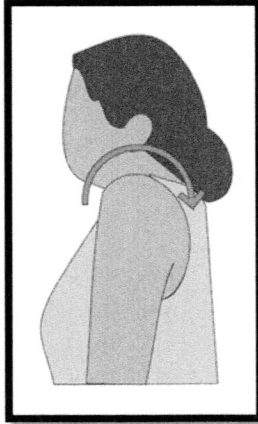

Stand tall with chin parallel to the floor and shoulders facing forward. Take your shoulders forward. Start rotating the shoulders taking them up and behind. Get your shoulder-blades together as you move the shoulders behind. Get shoulders back to the start position.

3.   Shoulder Forward Rotations:

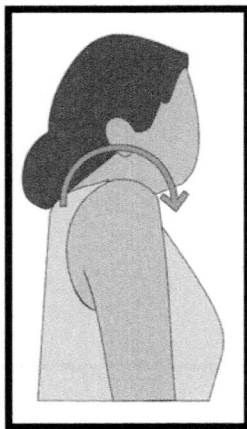

Stand tall with chin parallel to the floor and shoulders facing forward. Take your shoulders behind, getting your shoulder blades together. Continue rotating the shoulders taking them up and forwards. Get shoulders back to the start position. Repeat this sequence 10 times.

4.   Chest Expansions:

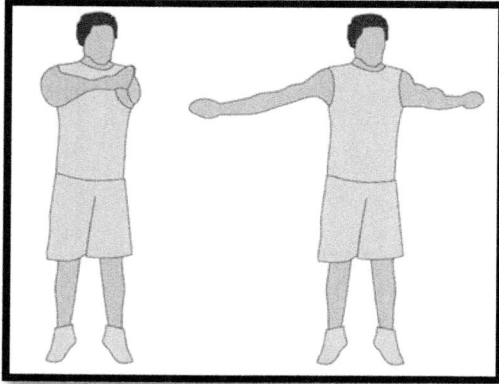

Stand tall with chin parallel to the floor and shoulders facing forward. Raise your arms to the shoulder level and take them back opening the chest. Repeat 10 times.

5.   Torso Rotations:

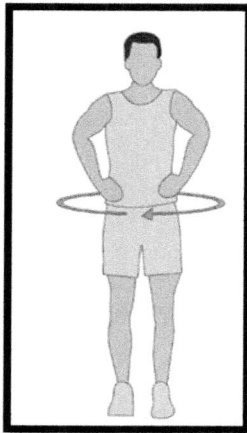

Stand tall with feet hip width distance apart. Place your hands on the waist and rotate your trunk clockwise. Repeat 10 times. Then rotate your trunk anti-clockwise. Repeat 10 times.

6.   Arm Rotations:

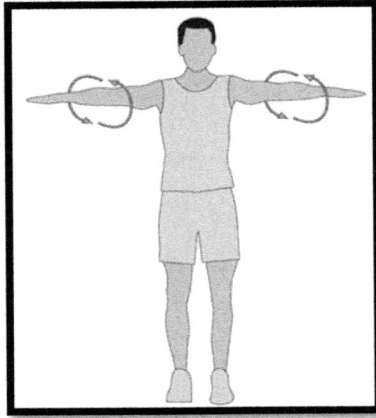

Stand tall with your feet hip width distance apart. Raise your arms to the side at shoulder level. Make circles with your arms moving them clockwise and anti-clockwise (10 times in each direction).

7.   Side Arm Raises:

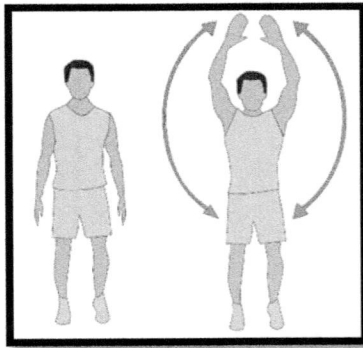

Stand tall with your feet hip width distance apart. Raise your both arms sideways up 10 times.

8.   Hip Rotation

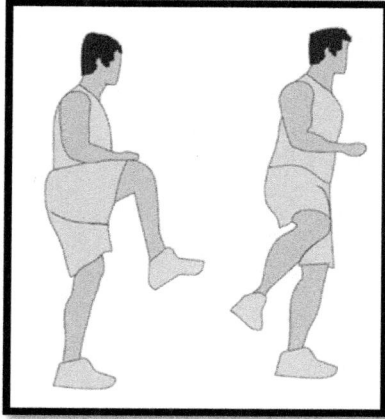

Lift your right leg and balance your body on the left foot. Rotate your leg at the hips in clockwise direction 10 times. Next rotate it in reverse direction 10 times. Repeat with the other leg.

9.   Jog on Spot

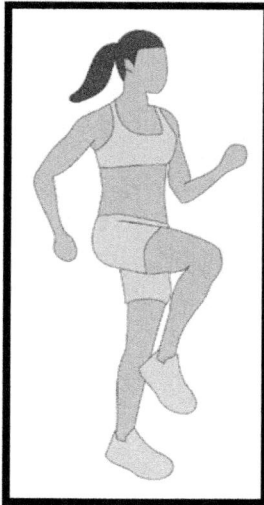

Jog on the spot. Try to lift your legs high enough to make your thighs parallel to the ground. Do 20 jogs of each foot.

10. Side to Side Hop

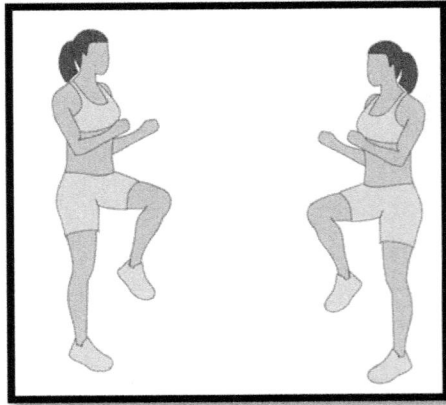

Balance yourself on one foot with the other leg raised high. Hop on the raised leg side, bringing that one down and raising the other leg up simultaneously. Repeat this 20 times.

Warm-up Sets: Every exercise you want to perform should begin with a warm up set. Warm up set includes all the exercises you are going to do, with little or no resistance for 10-15 repetitions with slower than normal tempo. So if you are working with a red band, you should do the warm-up with a green band.

UPPER BODY EXERCISES

Triceps Extension

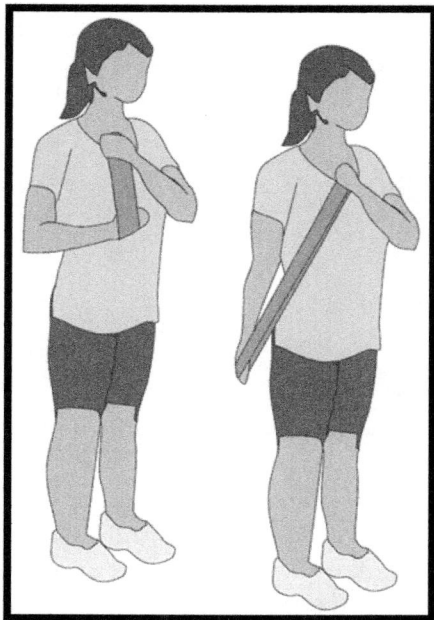

Stand tall with back straight and feet shoulder width apart. Hold one end of the band in hammer grip in left hand and brace it against your left collar bone. Hold the other end of the band in your right hand against your chest with open hand grip. Keeping your right elbow tucked in by the side of your trunk, push your right arm to full extension. Make sure that the left hand stays in a braced position at your chest. Do required number of repetitions. Repeat on the other side.

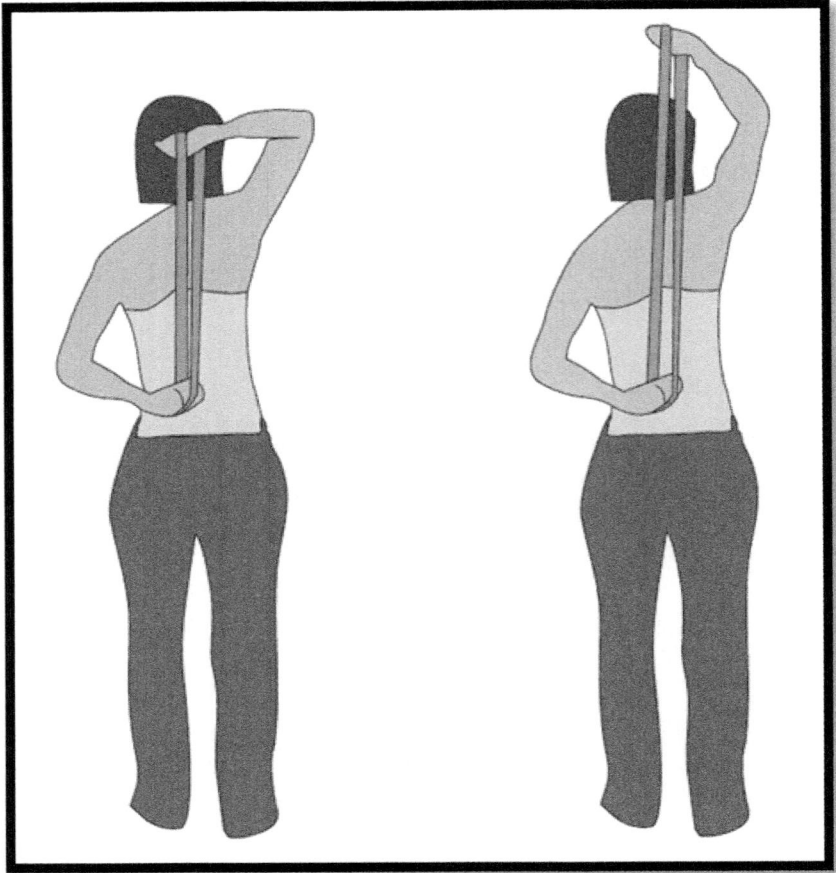

Stand tall with back straight and feet shoulder width apart. Raise right elbow to forehead level and hold one end of the resistance loop in right hand with up grip. Drop the other end of the resistance loop behind your back and hold it with the left hand (hand facing out). Maintain this level throughout the exercise. Extend the right elbow (but do not lock the elbow) and pull the band out. The right hand is moving up and out. Do the required number of repetitions. Repeat on the other side.

Horizontal Arm Extension

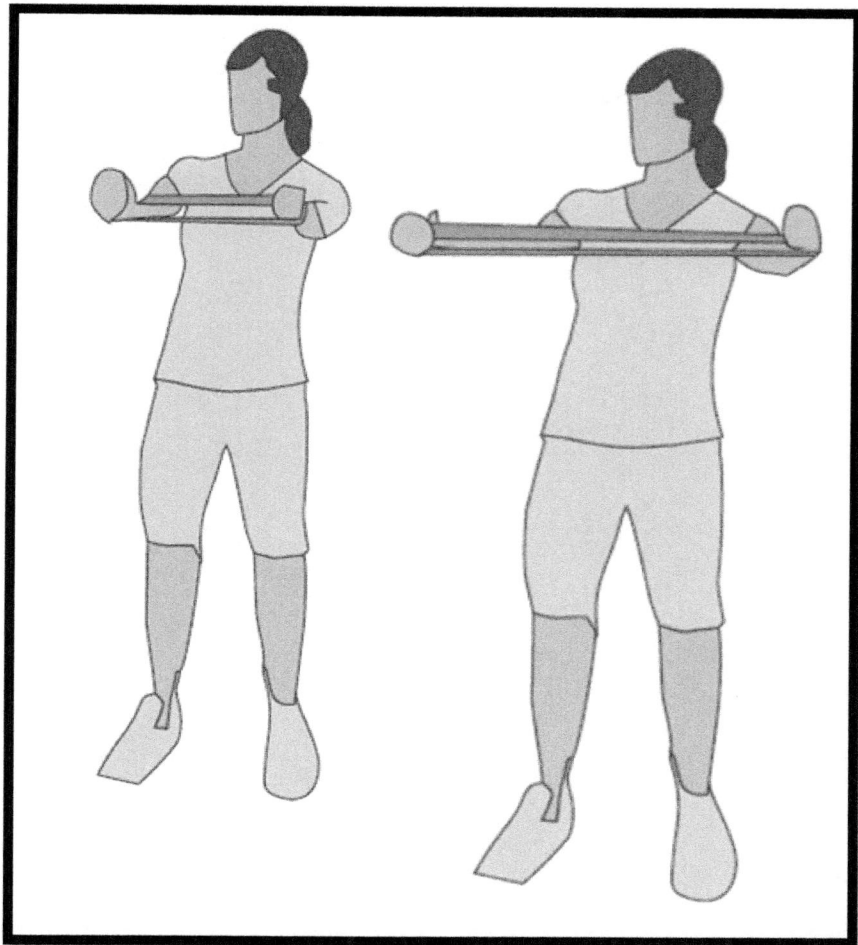

Stand tall with back straight and feet shoulder width apart. Place the resistance band around your wrists and extend your arms in front of you at shoulder level, hands shoulder width apart. Keeping arms slightly bent at elbows, pull the band apart by applying outward pressure to your forearms. Move the arms horizontally maintaining them at shoulder level. Hold the stretched position for 5 seconds. Release the stretch and return to the start position. Do required number of repetitions.

Vertical Arm Extension

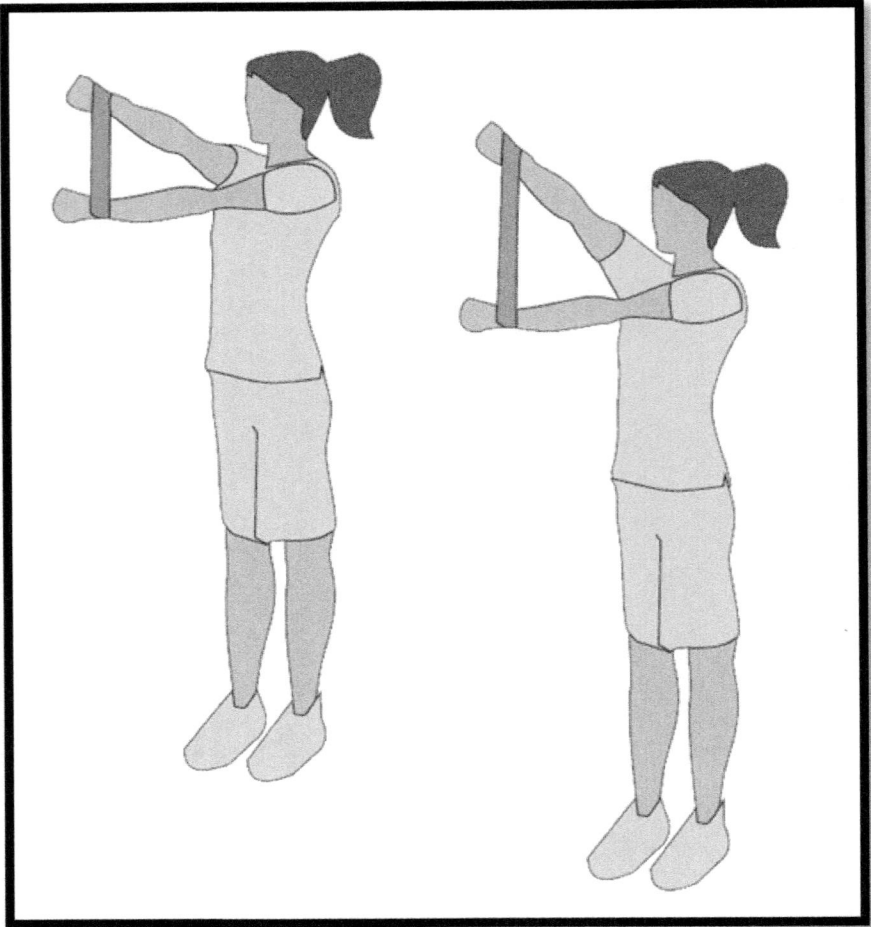

Stand tall with your back straight and feet shoulder width apart. Stretch arms in front of you, with left arm at shoulder level and right arm above it. Keeping your arms slightly bent at elbows, pull the band apart by applying upward pressure to right forearm and downward pressure to left forearm. The arms move in the vertical plane. Hold the stretched position for 5 seconds. Return to the start position. Switch the arms and repeat. Do required number of repetitions.

Rear Arm Extension

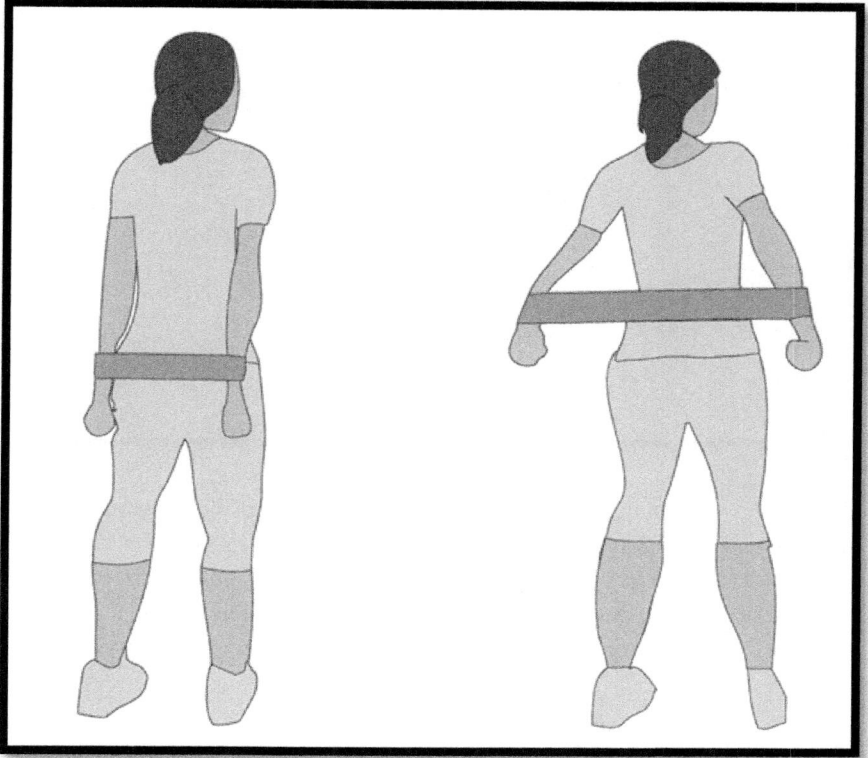

Stand tall with back straight and feet shoulder width apart. Place the resistance band around your wrists and hold your arm behind you. Keeping your arms slightly bent, pull the band apart by applying outward pressure to your forearms. Your arms move in horizontal plane. Hold the stretched position for 5 counts. Return to the start position and repeat.

Bicep Curl

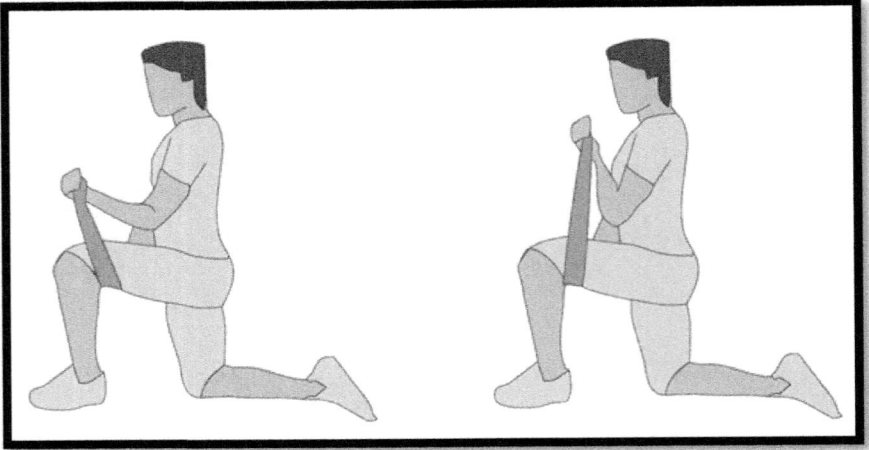

Do a lunge with right knee touching the ground. Loop the resistance band around your left knee, and hold the other end in your left hand with up grip. Keeping your back tall and abdomen tucked in, curl the arm at elbow, pulling the band up. Squeeze the biceps tightly in the fully contracted position. Slowly lower to the start position. Repeat on the other side.

Internal Rotation

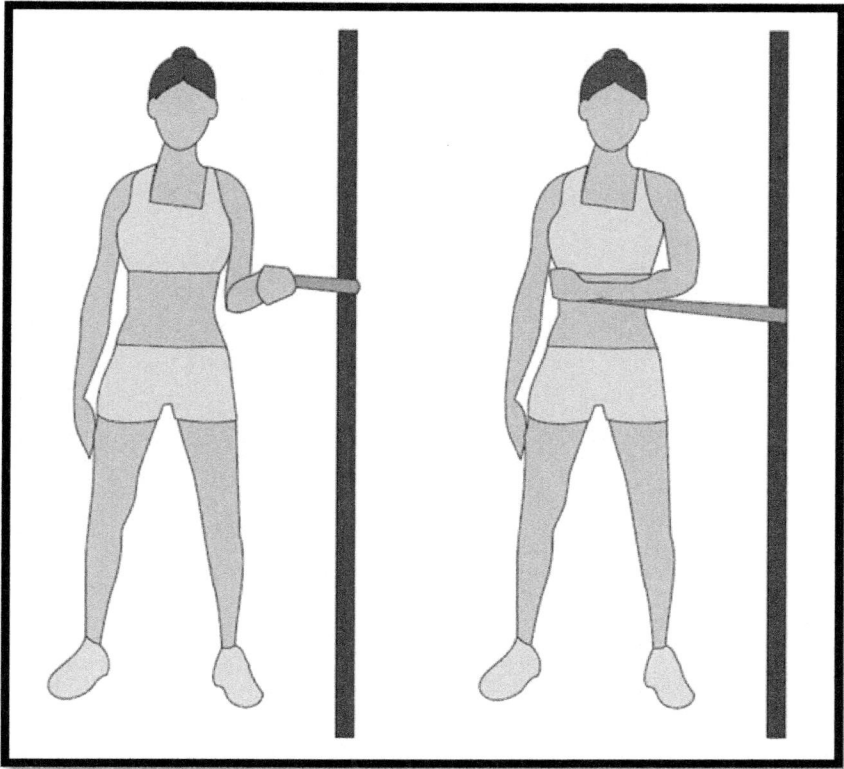

Stand tall, abdomen tucked in, gluteus tight and feet hip width distance apart. Loop the resistance band through a support (like the window rail). Hold the other end of the band in hammer grip, keeping arm tucked by side of the trunk and forearm at 90 degrees to the upper arm, parallel to the floor. Pull the band inward, taking forearm horizontally to the abdomen. Hold the stretched position for 5 counts and release. Bring forearm back to the start position. Repeat with the other arm.

External Rotation

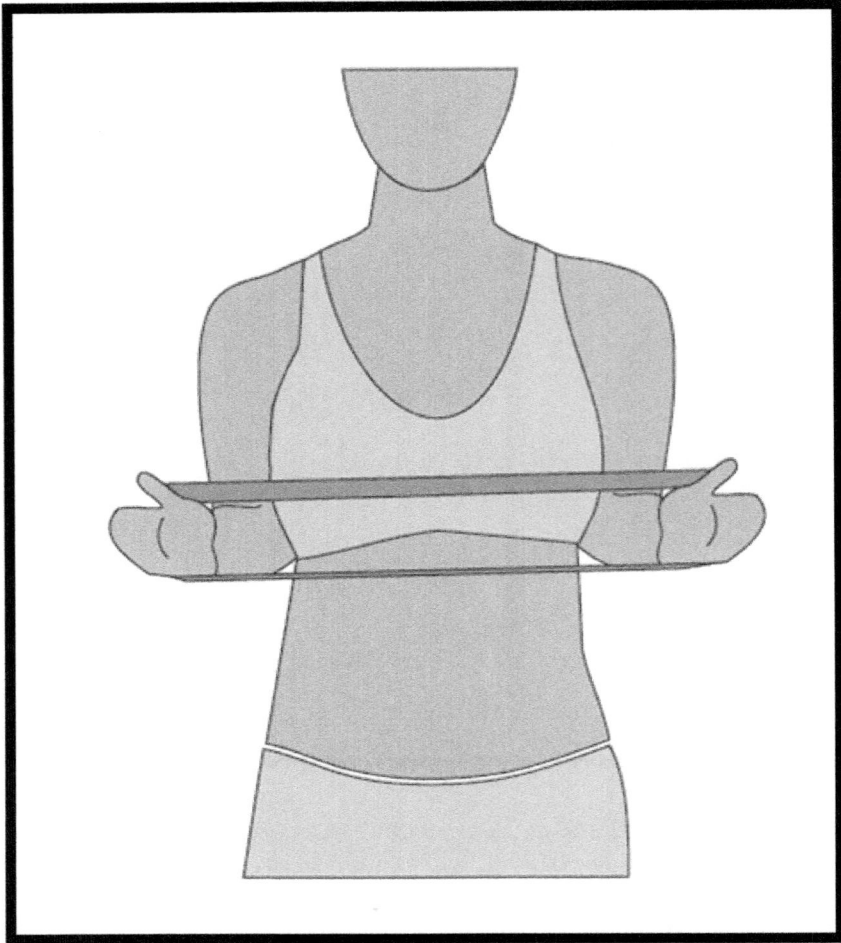

Stand tall, with back straight, abdomen tucked in and feet hip width distance apart. Hold the resistance loop in open hand grip with both hands, with elbows tucked by side of the trunk and forearms at 90 degrees to the arm. Pull the band horizontally outwards, moving the hands apart, keeping your elbows tucked in by side of the trunk. Hold the stretched position for 5 counts and release. Come back to the start position.

Hand Scrunches

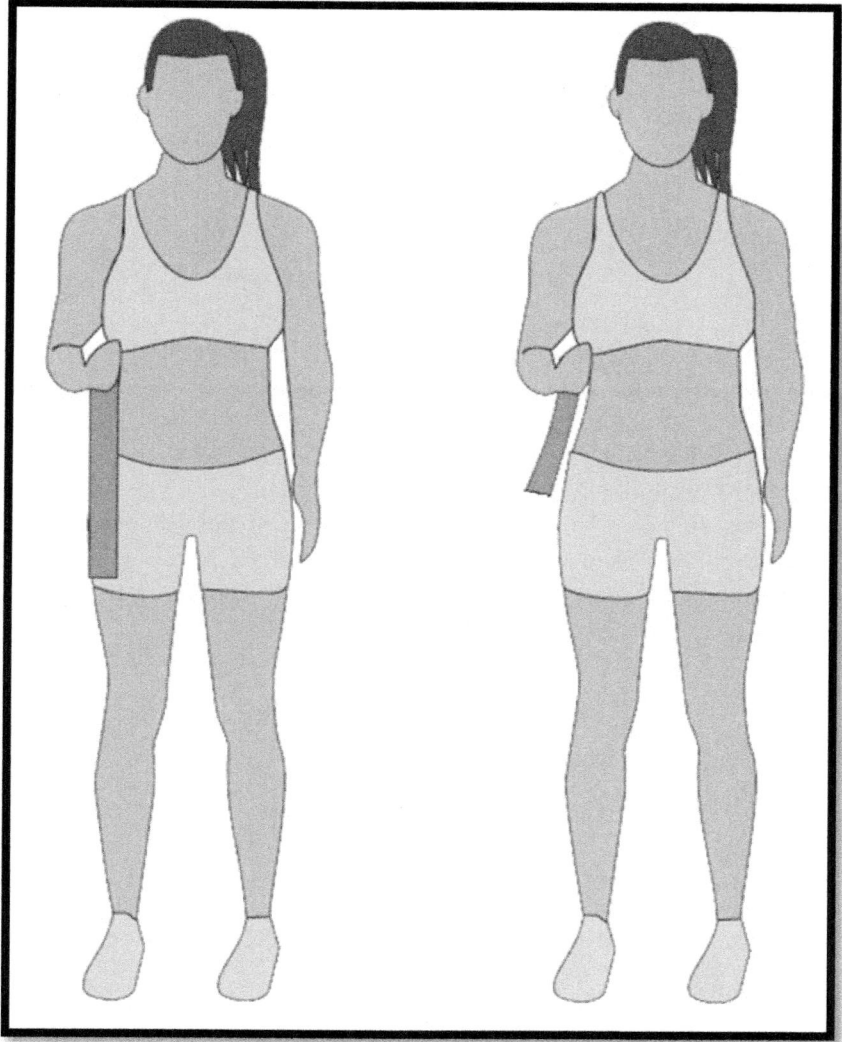

Scrunch the band in your hand and release. Repeat it 10 times.

Bear Crawls

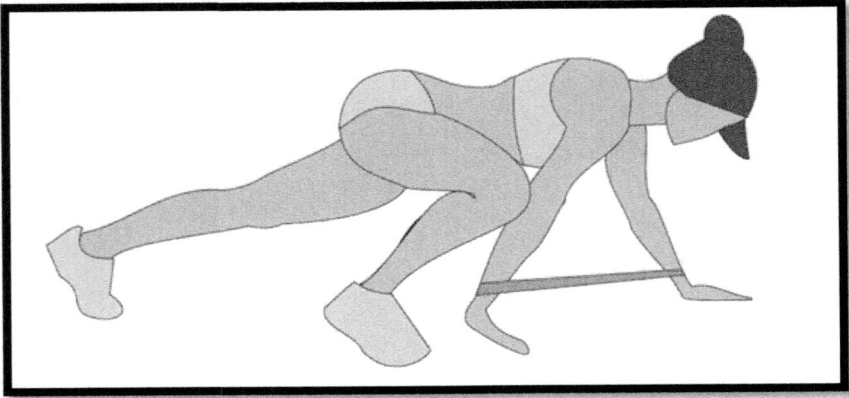

Put the resistance band around your wrists and come in all fours position with your hands under the shoulder and knees under the hips. Start crawling, moving your left hand and right leg forward and vice-versa, maintaining shoulders and hips in one horizontal plane. Always maintain tension in the loop band. You can move forwards, sidewards and backwards to have variation in the exercise.

Lateral Arm Raise (Rotator Cuff)

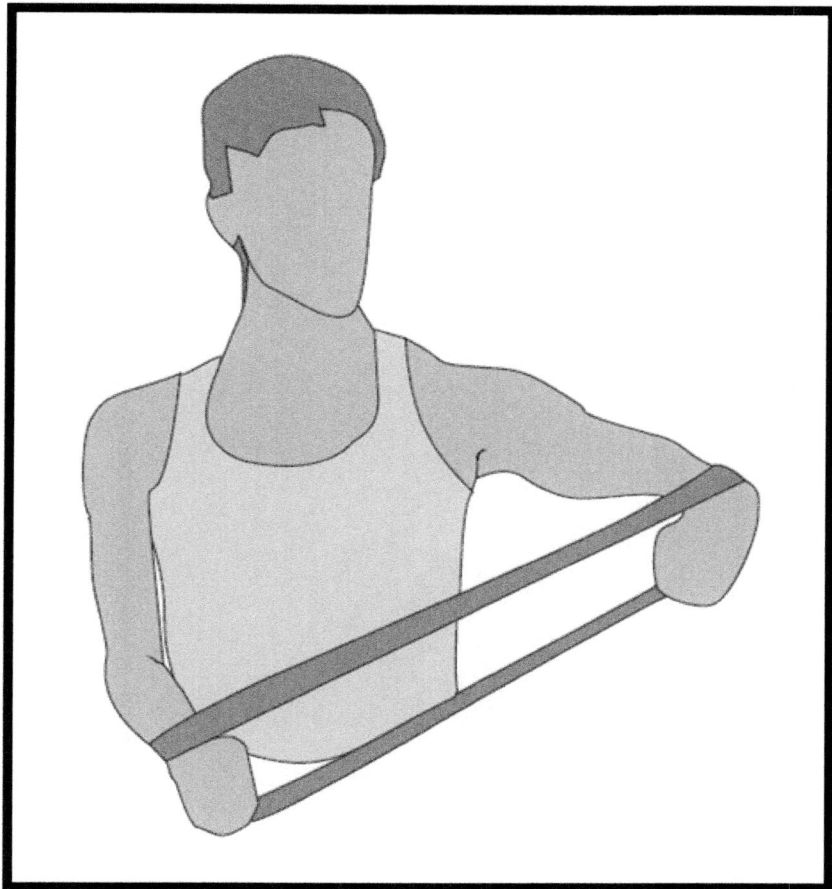

Stand tall with back straight, abdomen tucked in and feet hip width distance apart. Bend the arms to 90 degrees at the elbows and tuck them by the side of your trunk. Place the resistance band around your wrists. Putting outward pressure on both the ends of the band, raise your left arm laterally upwards, maintaining the 90 degree bend at elbow. Hold the left arm in fully stretched position for 5 counts. Release the stretch slowly, getting left arm back to the starting position. Repeat on the right side.

Seated Concentration Curl

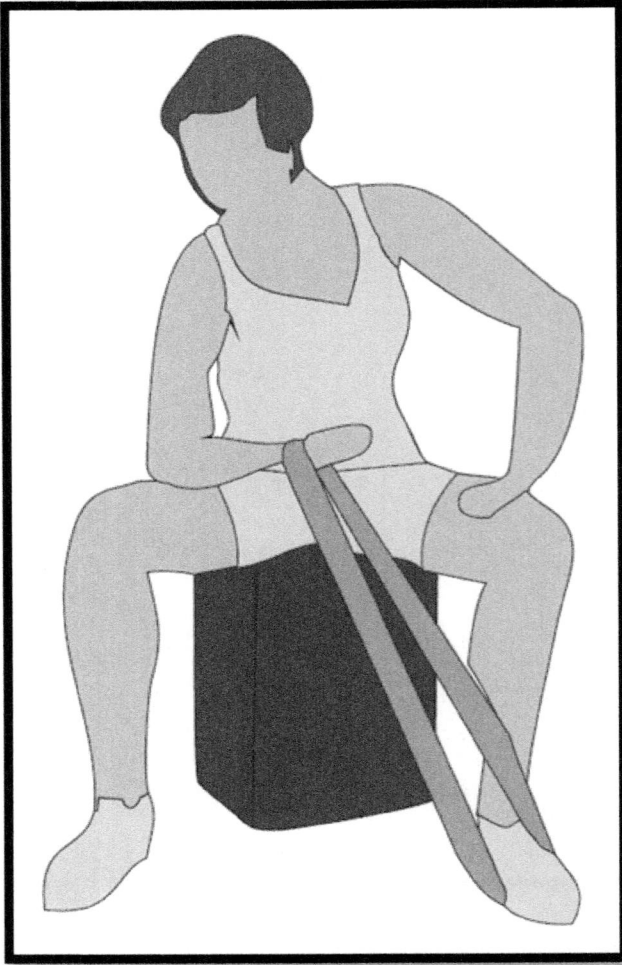

Sit on a stool, placing resistance loop over one foot and grasp the band with an up grip in your right hand. Sit with your abdomen tucked in and bend your elbow to bring the band towards your chest. There should be no movement through the upper torso. Squeeze the biceps at the fully contracted position. Return to the start position slowly. Do the required number of repetitions. Repeat on the other side.

Wrist Curl

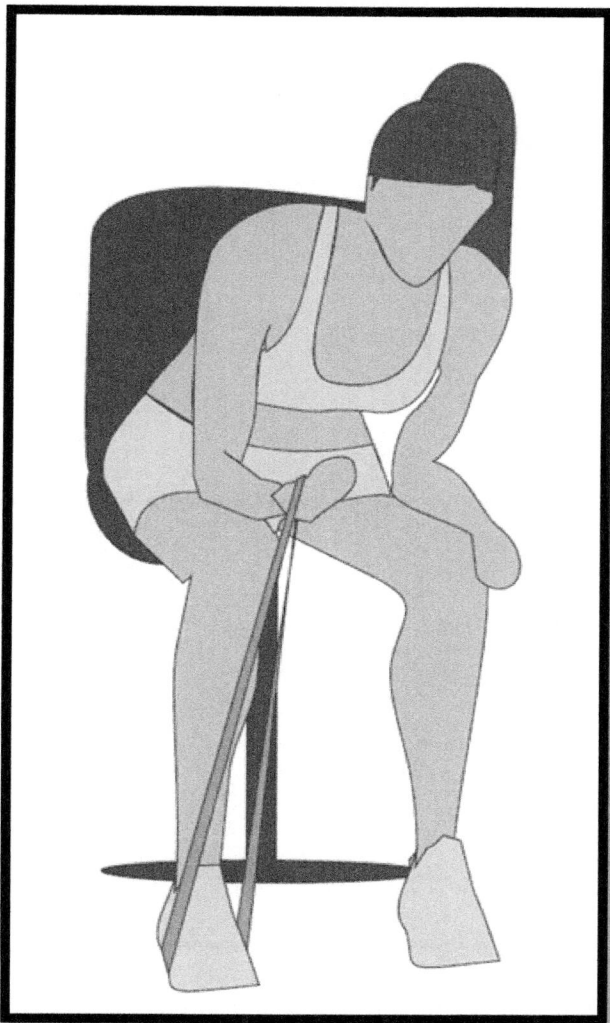

Put the resistance band over your foot and hold the band in your hand in up grip with your forearm resting on the thighs. Sit on the chair with your knees and ankle at 90 degrees, hip width distance apart. Bend your wrist, pulling the band up. The movement should be slow and rhythmic. Feel the muscles of your front forearm contracting. Do the required number of repetitions. Repeat on the other side.

LOWER BODY EXERCISES

Bridge Thrust

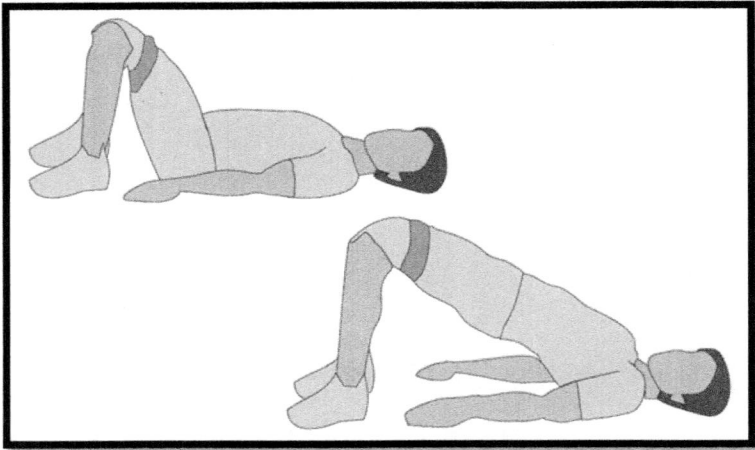

Lie down straight on your back with legs bent at knee, feet flat on the floor, shoulder width apart and hands by the side of your body. Place the resistance band around your thighs, just above the knees. Exhale and imprint your back on the floor. Inhale and raise your hips up till your back, hips and thighs come in one line. Hold this position for 5 seconds (keep breathing as you hold the position). Slowly release the position and get your hips down back to the start position as you exhale. Keep tension in the loop band throughout the exercise. Repeat.

Side Step Squats

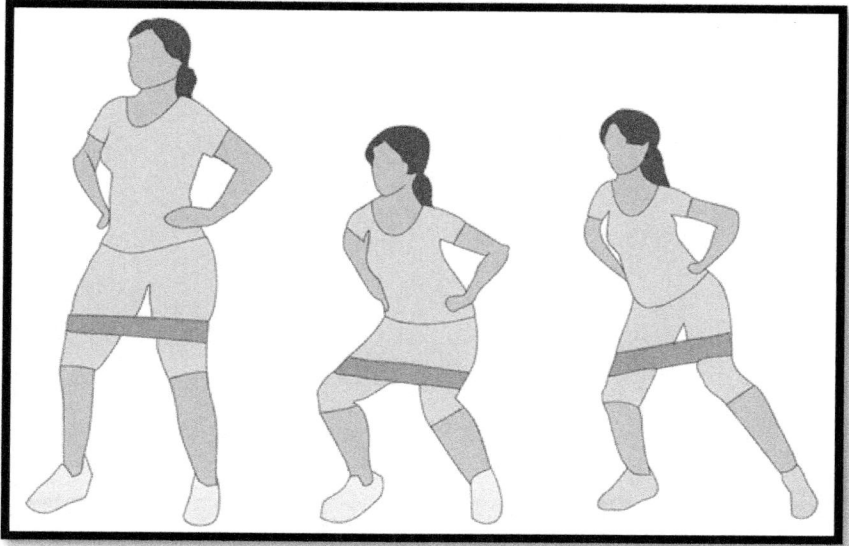

Loop the resistance band around your lower thigh just above the knees. Stand with feet shoulder width apart. Move the left leg horizontally sidewards as if taking a side step. Go in squat position and hold there for 5 seconds. Release the stretch and come back to start position. Repeat it on the right side.

Lying Hip Abduction

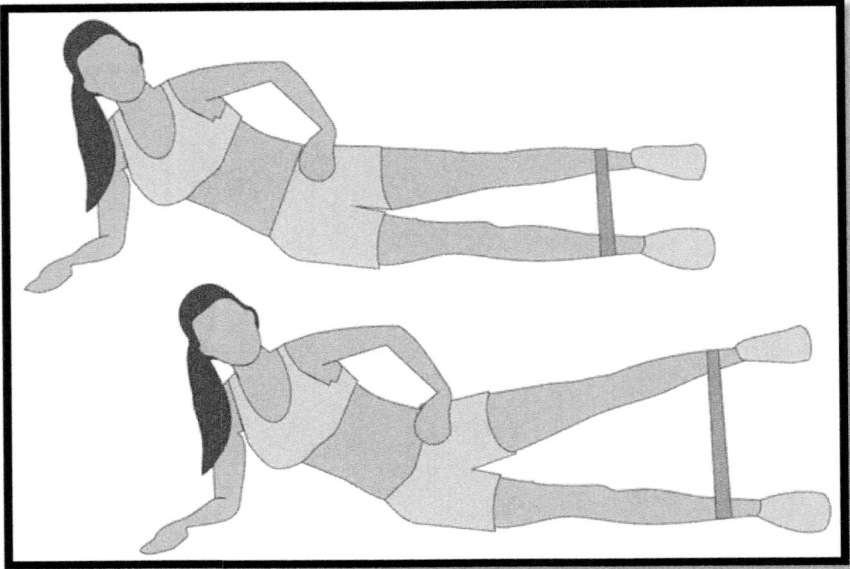

Put the resistance loop around your ankles. Lie on your right side, supporting your torso on the bent right arm. Your upper leg is above your lower leg, hip width apart. Raise your left leg up, pulling the resistance band. Hold the left leg at maximum stretch position for 5 counts (without changing the form). Slowly lower the left leg to start position. Repeat on the other side.

Lying Leg Raise

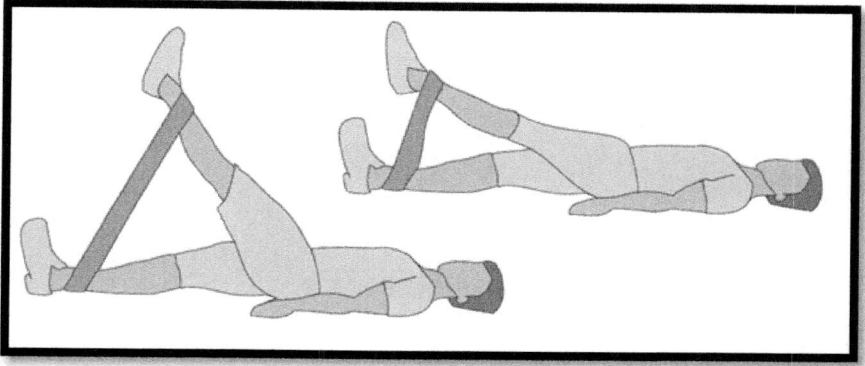

Put the resistance loop around your ankle. Lie down on your back with one leg over the other and arms by the side of your body. Tuck your abdominals in as you exhale. Inhale and lift your upper leg up, to the maximum stretch position. Hold the leg up for 5 counts. Keep breathing. Exhale and slowly get the leg down to start position. Repeat with other leg.

Standing Hip Abduction

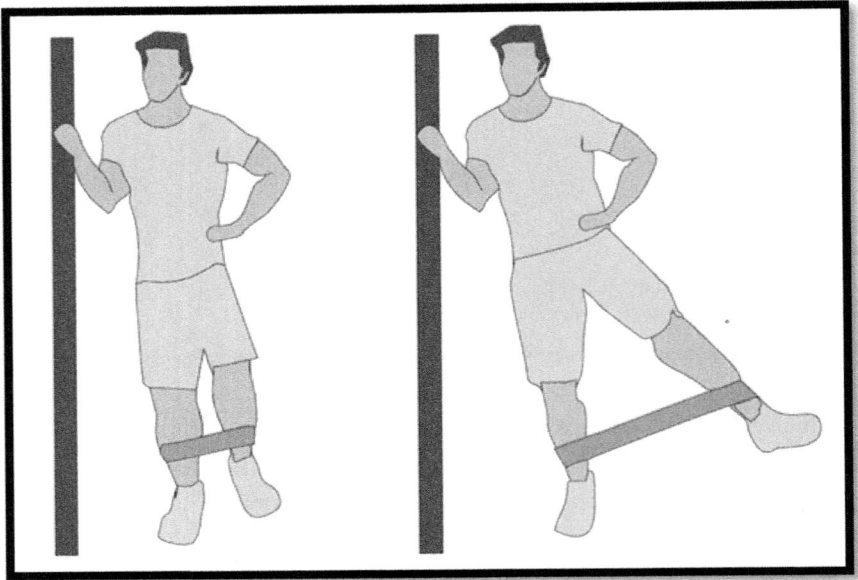

Put the resistance loop around your ankle. Stand tall with the right side of your body against the wall and feet hip width distance apart. Squeeze your right glutes and stand on the right foot. Start raising your left leg sideways upwards pulling the resistance loop apart. Feel your left abductors contracting. Hold your leg up in maximum stretch position for 5 counts. Slowly lower the leg down to start position. Perform the required number of repetitions and then repeat with the other leg.

Band Squats

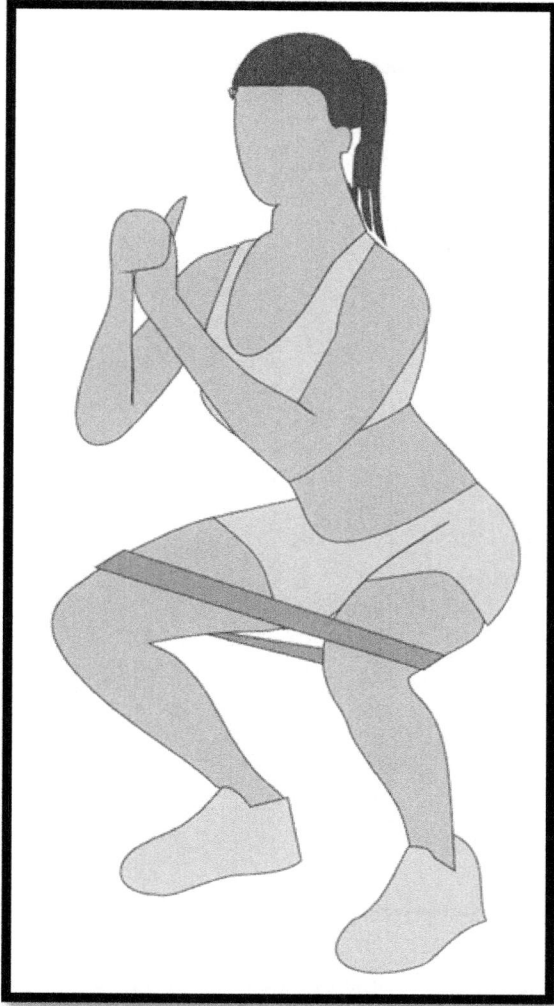

Stand with your resistance loop around your thighs, just above the knees. Move your feet shoulder width apart, with chest and head up. Sit your hips back bending at the knee. Push your knees out and against the resistance loop as you squat, getting your thighs parallel to the floor. Once your thighs are parallel to the floor, push through your heels and come up to the starting position. Repeat.

Leg Extension

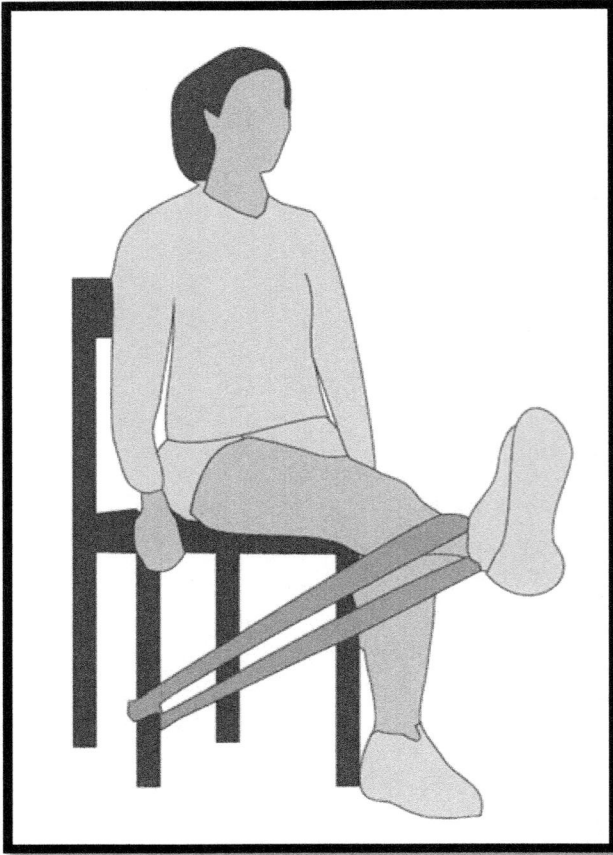

Sit tall on the chair, with abdomen tucked in, feet hip width distance apart and flat on the ground. Place one end of the band in leg of the chair to lock it and other end over your right ankle. Hold the base of the chair with your hands as you raise the right leg against the resistance of the band. Contract your front thigh muscle as you raise the leg and hold the lower leg in line with thigh. Hold the leg in this position for 5 counts. Slowly lower the leg down to the start position. Perform the required number of repetitions and then repeat with the other leg.

Clam Shell

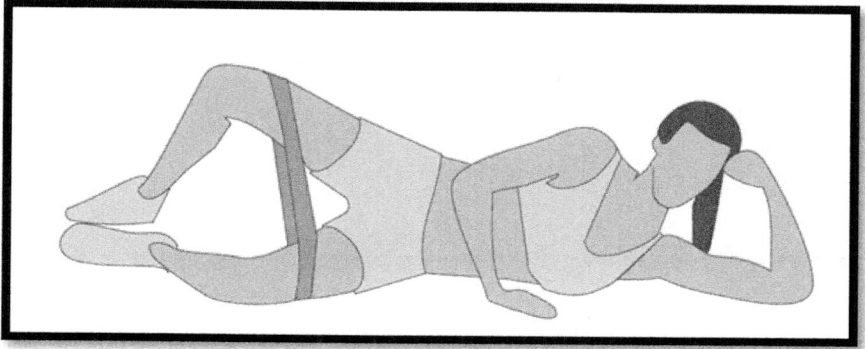

Slide the resistance loop above the knees. Lie in the side lying position, with your right knee above the left, your right feet above the left, hips and knees at 90 degrees and ankles touching each other. Your upper body is supported by right hand placed flat in front of the upper body. Keeping your feet together raise your right knee up (taking right leg in external rotation), without moving the pelvis and keeping left leg still. Pause at the top for a second and slowly move the right knee down to the starting position. After required number of repetitions, repeat on the left side.

Supinated Clamshell

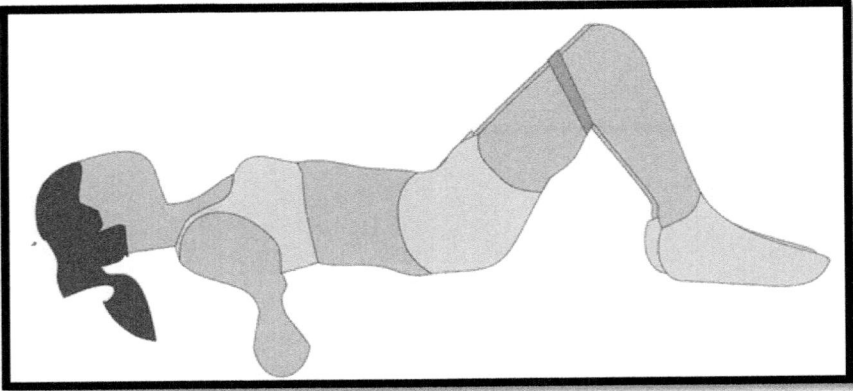

Put the resistance loop around your thighs just above the knees. Lie down on your back with hips and knees flexed (knees flexed at 90 degrees) and abdomen tucked in. The knees and feet should be hip width distance apart. Pull the knees apart while contracting your glutes for 2-3 seconds. Slowly come back to the starting position. Perform the required number of repetitions.

Thigh Thrust

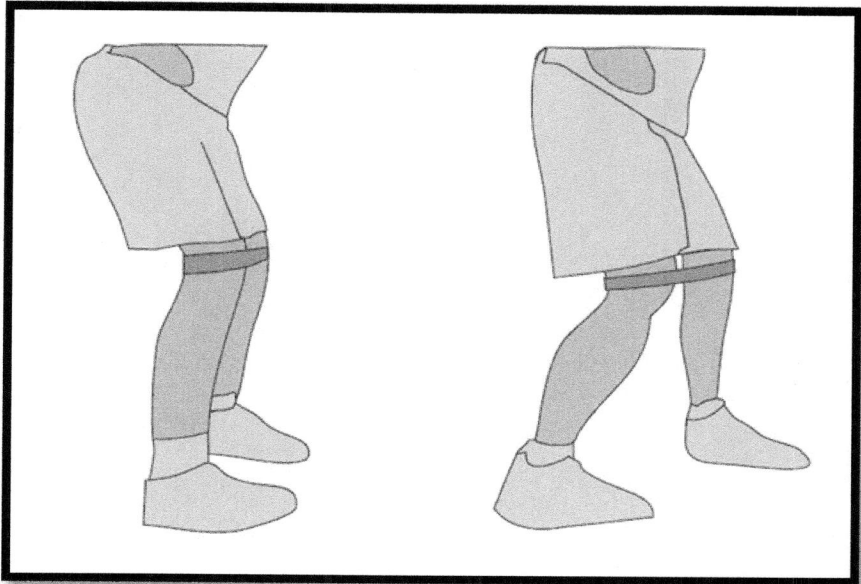

Loop the resistance band above your knees and stand with feet hip width distance apart. The band should be stretched. Resist the pull of the band as you take five steps forward. Continue to resist the pull of the band as you take five steps back. You can repeat this exercise walking sideways.

Lateral Walk

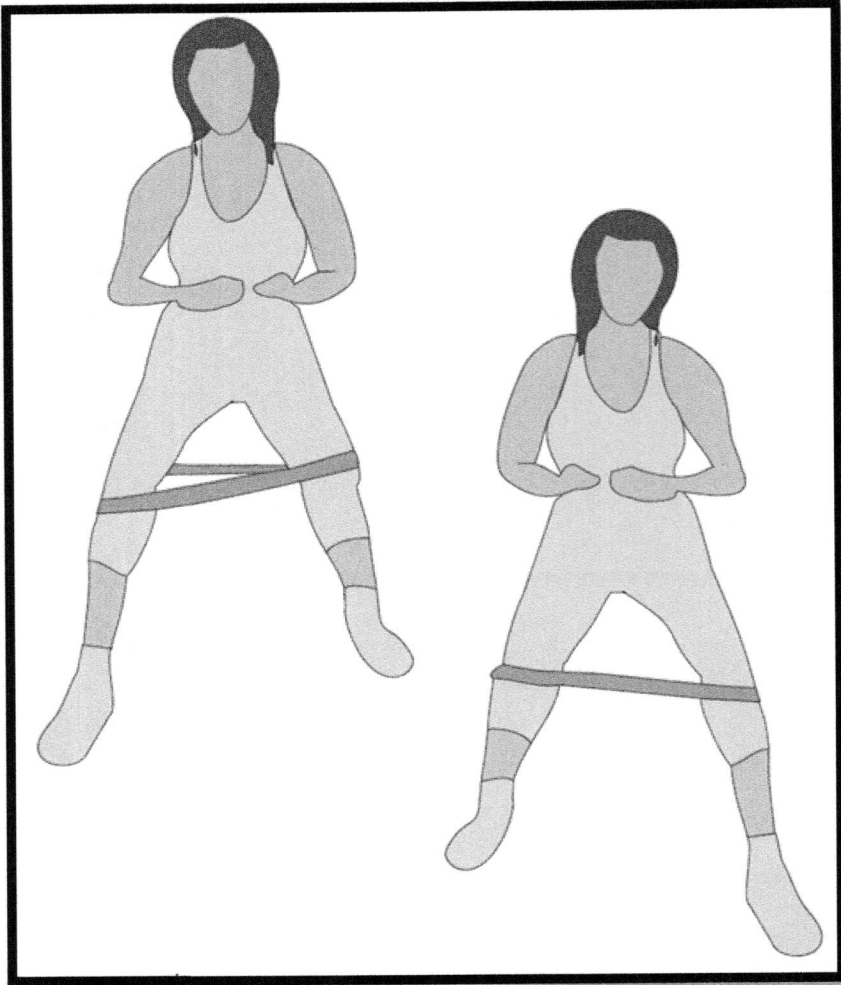

Stand with feet shoulder width apart and resistance loop band around the lower thigh, just above the knees. Create tension in the band. Bend at your knees, keeping the back tall. Take an exaggerated step to the right to maximally stretch out the loop band. Continue in that direction for 5 steps. Take five exaggerated steps to the left to return to the start position. Repeat on the other side.

Standing Hip Flexion

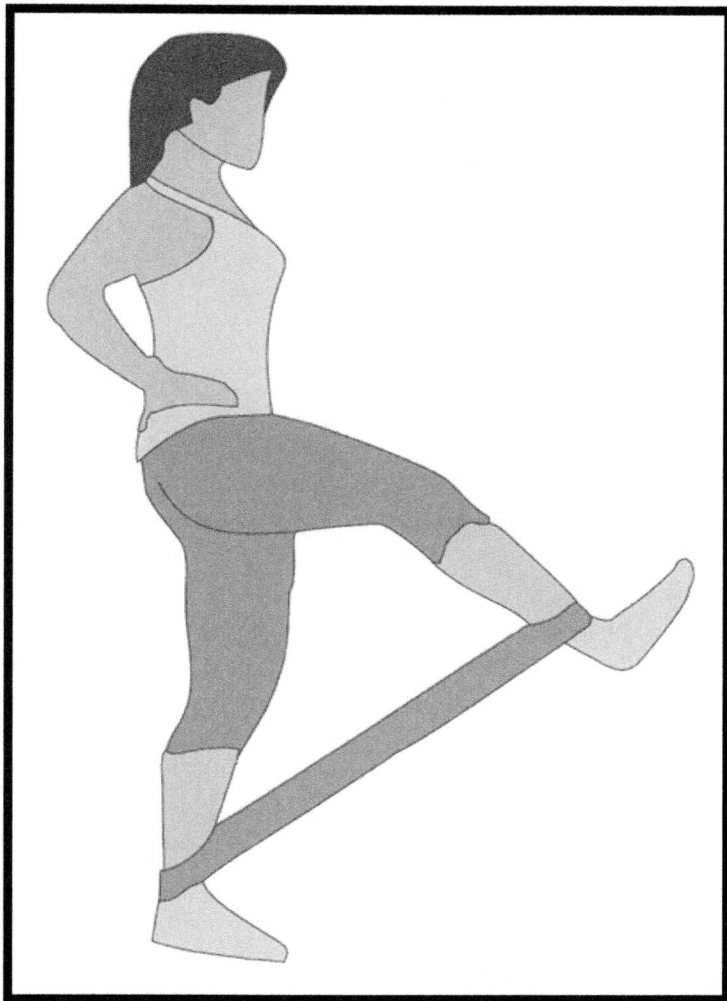

Stand tall with feet hip width distance apart and the resistance loop band around the ankles. Shifting your weight to the left leg, raise your right leg forward, pulling the band. Keep your torso tall all the time. Never lock (hyperextend) the knees. Perform required repetitions. Repeat on the other side.

Single Leg Loop Bridge

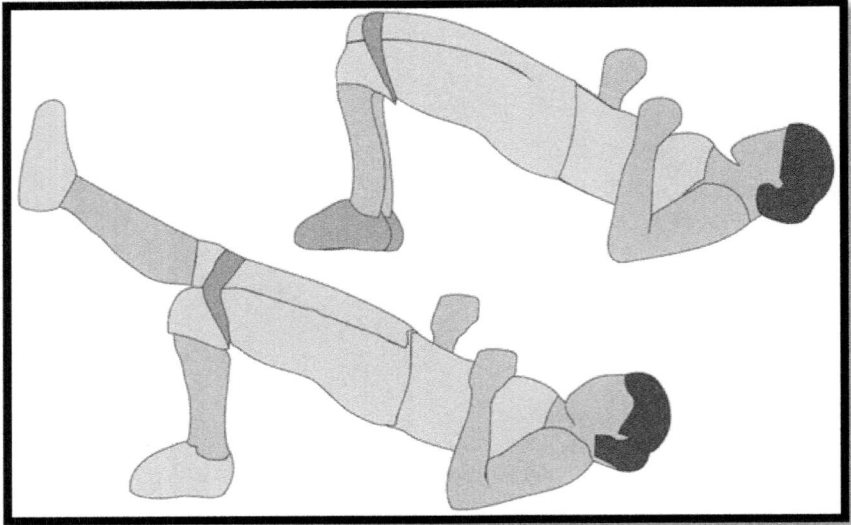

Loop the resistance band around your lower thigh, just above the knees. Lie down in bridge position (feet flat on the floor, hand palms down by your sides, abdomen braced and hips lifted up with glutes contracted). Raise your right leg up, keeping thigh in line with thigh and pull your toes towards you. Hold this position for 5 counts. Slowly lower down the leg to start position. Perform required number of times. Repeat on the other side.

Hamstring Curls

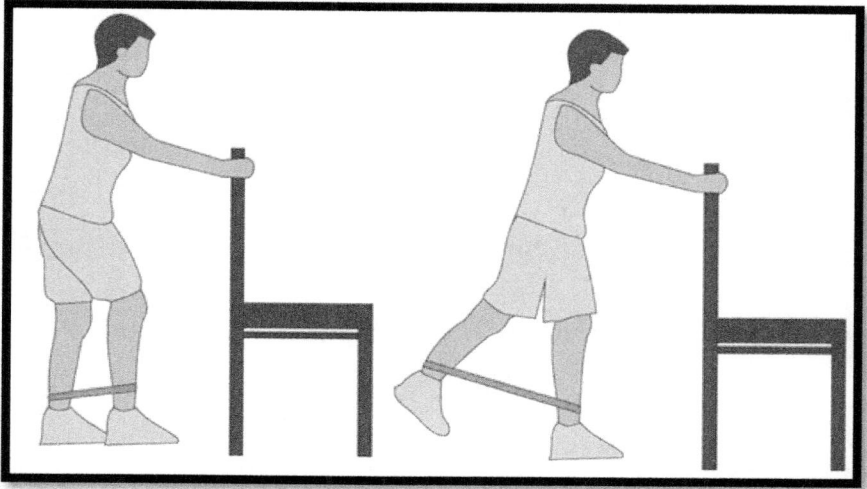

Stand tall with feet hip width distance apart, facing a chair and put one or both hand on the chair to balance. Put the resistance loop band around your ankles. You may put one end of the loop around right ankle and other end under the left heel to stabilize it. Shift your weight to left leg keeping your abdominals engaged and buttocks contracted. Bend your right leg at knee, stretching the band to maximum. Keep your torso tall all the time. Slowly get the right leg back to the start position. Perform the required number of repetitions. Repeat on the other side.

Standing Hip Adduction

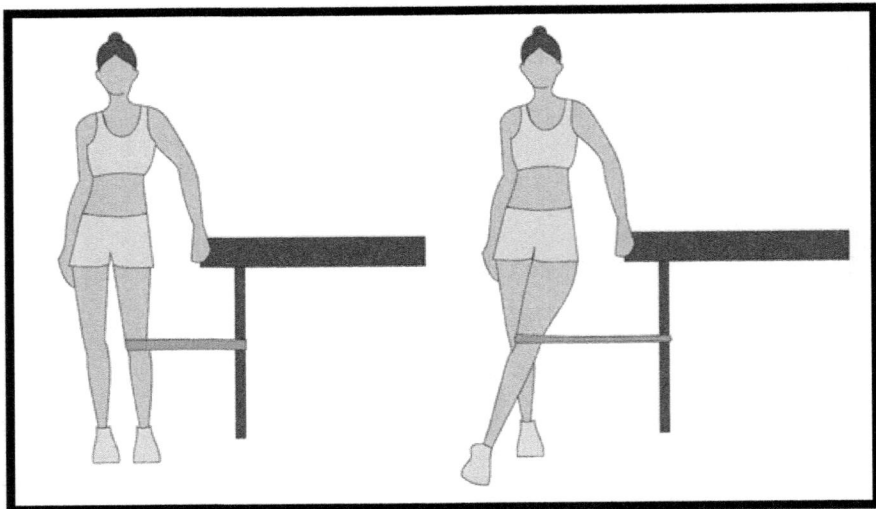

Stand tall by the side of a table or pole (around 1 feet away from it) with your abdomen tucked in and feet hip width distance apart. Loop the band around the ankle of the leg near to table/pole and the leg of the table/pole. You can hold onto the furniture or the wall to maintain balance while taking the leg sidewards, away from the table/pole. With your toes pointing forwards and keeping your leg straight, lift your leg out to the side till it comes off the ground. Return to the start position. Perform the required number of repetitions. Repeat on the other side.

Standing Hip Extension

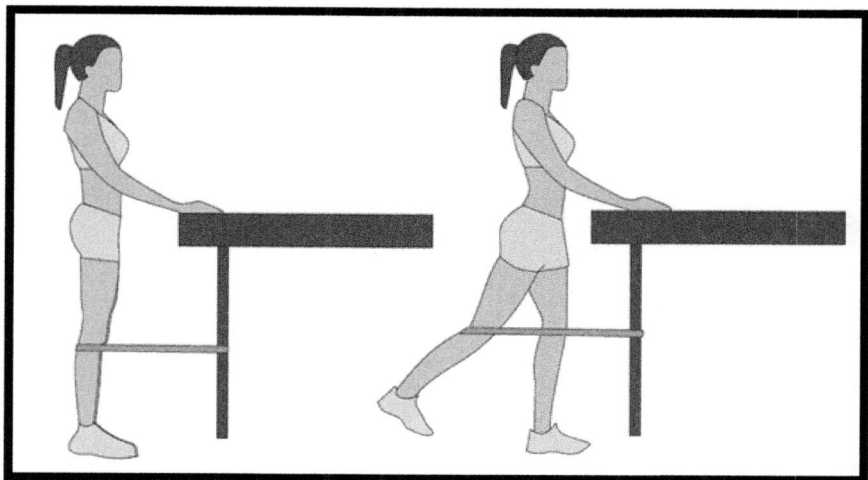

Loop the band around your right leg and the leg of a table or a pole. Stand tall facing the table, with your abdomen tucked in and feet hip width distance apart. You can hold onto the furniture or wall to maintain the balance, as you raise your right leg. Keeping your leg straight and toes pointing forwards, push your leg backwards till it comes slightly above the ground. Return to the start position. Perform the required number of repetitions. Repeat on the other side.

Seated Leg Extension

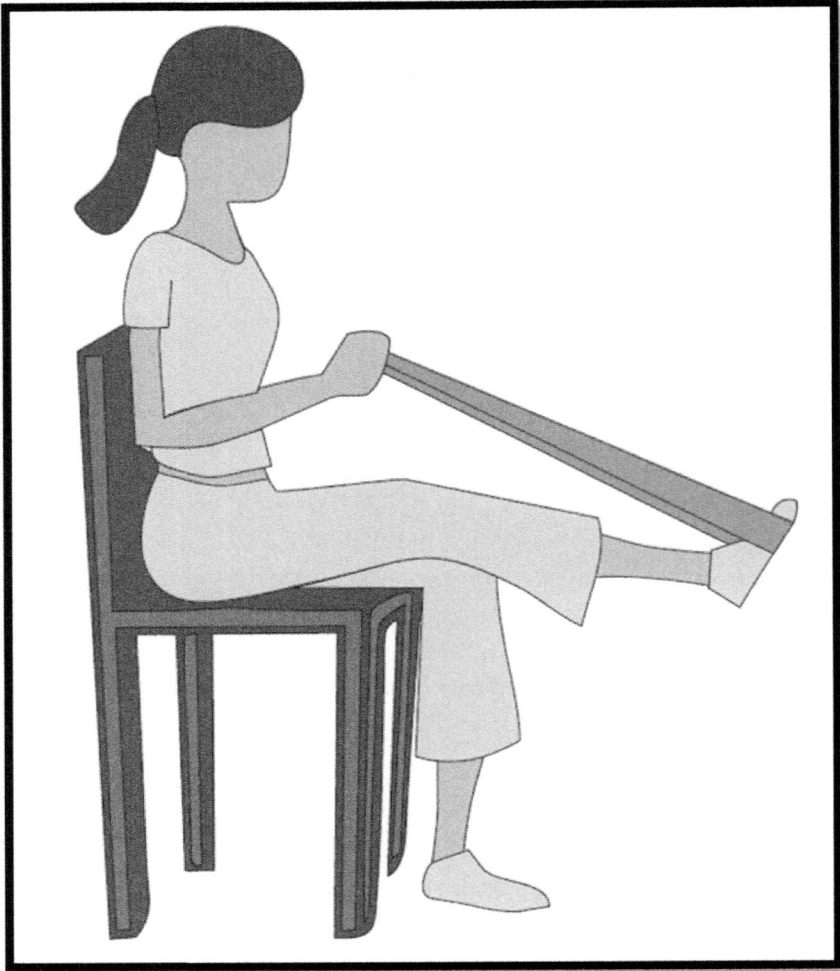

Sit on the chair with back tall and supported. Put the loop band around your right foot. Hold the band in the right hand and extend your leg against the resistance of loop band. Hold for 5 counts and releases. Perform required number of repetitions on each leg.

Hip Seated Abduction

Loop the resistance band around mid of your thigh and sit tall on the chair. Push your legs out to the sides, so that the band stretches. Return to the start position. Perform required number of repetitions.

Glute Bridges

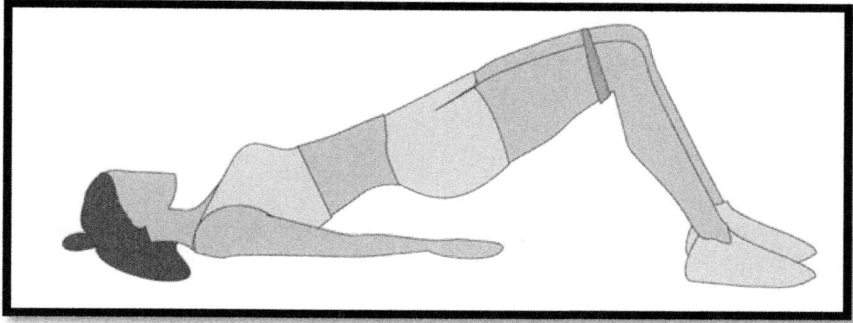

Loop the resistance band around your legs just above the knees. Lie down on your back with legs bent to 90 degrees at the knees and arms by the side of your body. Spread your legs little bit so that there is tension in the resistance loop band. Imprint your back as you exhale. Inhale, contract your glutes and raise your hips up till your knees, hips and back are in one line. Return back to the start position slowly as you exhale. Maintain the tension in the band. Perform required number of repetitions.

CHEST & BACK EXERCISES

Lateral Push Up / Band Walk

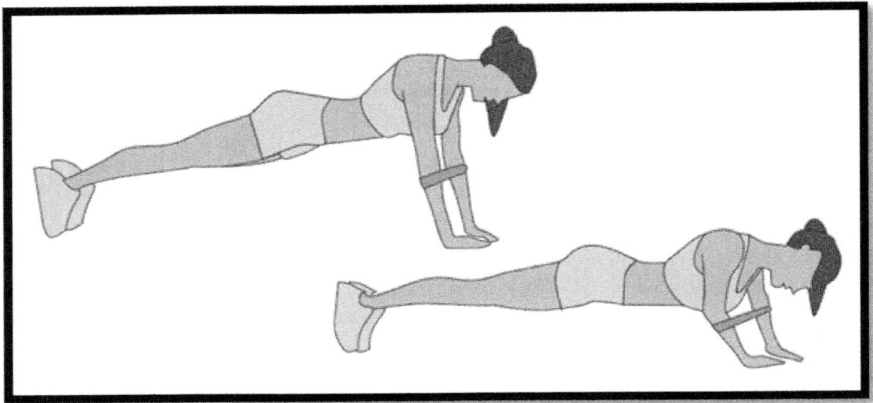

Come in plank position with arms extended and hands shoulder width apart. Put the resistance loop band around the arms. Go down on the hands, bending the arms at elbows, with the lateral side of arms pushing against the band. Hold this position for 5 counts and come back to the start position. Perform required number of repetitions.

Lateral Pull Down

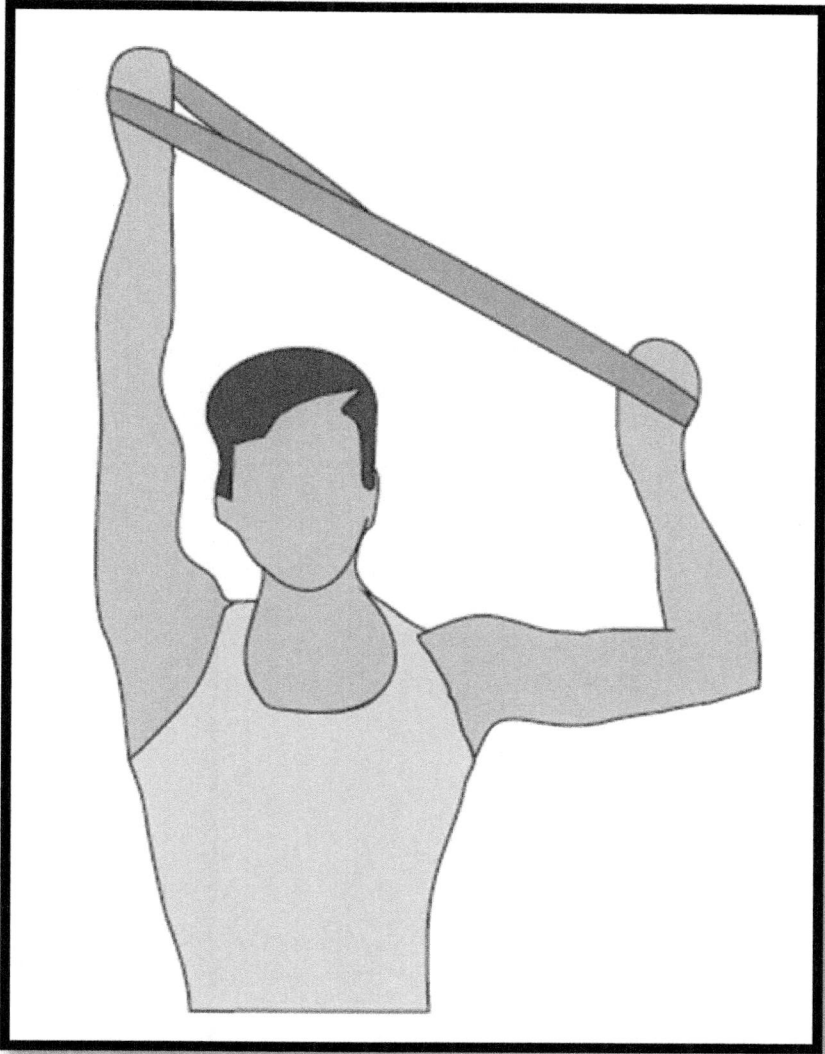

Hold the resistance loop band in down grip, with arms stretched overhead. Stand tall with your feet hip width distance apart. Keeping the right arm stretched up, start pulling the band laterally out and down with your left hand, engaging your back muscles. Hold the stretched position for 1 second and return slowly to the start position. Perform required number of repetitions. Repeat on the other side.

ABDOMINAL EXERCISES

Oblique Overhead Extension

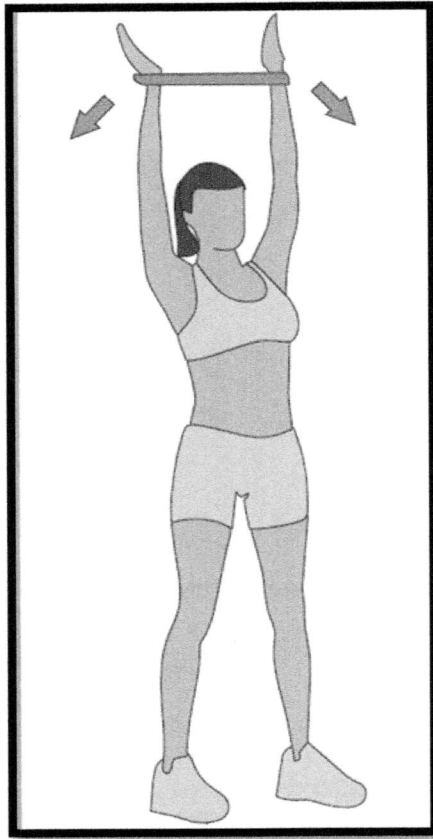

Stand tall with your feet shoulder feet apart and knees slightly bent. Stretch the arms overhead and hold the loop band in the open grip in your hands. Stretch the band out to keep it taut throughout the exercise. Bend to your right in a controlled manner and feel the stretch in your left obliques. Hold the stretch for 3 counts. Return to the start position. Repeat on the other side. Perform required number of bends.

Bicycles

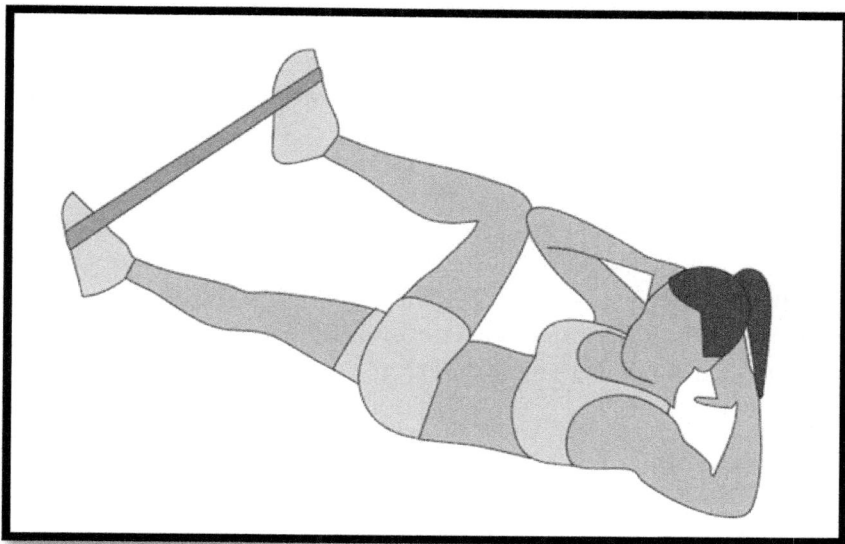

Loop the resistance band around your feet and lie down on your back. Place your hands behind your head. Raise both of your feet about one foot into the air. Pull your right knee towards the abdomen and get your left elbow towards the right knee in a crunching motion. Feel the contraction in your obliques as your elbow touches the knee. Slowly return to the start position and repeat on the other side.

Abdominal Crunch with Rotations

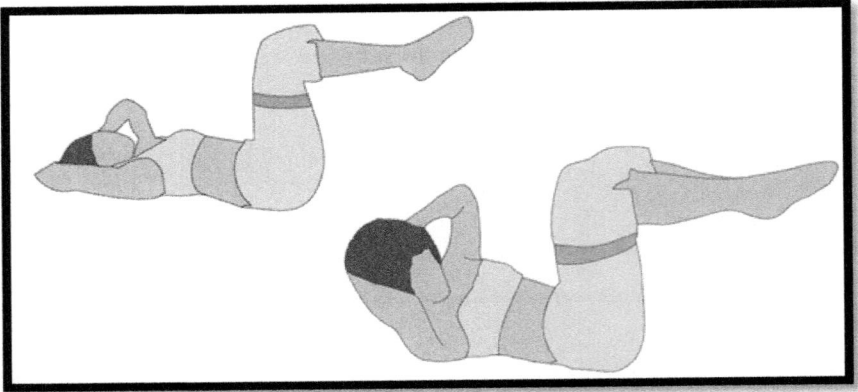

Lie down flat on your back with your legs bent to 90 degrees at hip and knees and your lower leg parallel to the floor. Put the loop band around mid-thigh and spread your legs little apart to make the band taut. Place your hands with fingers interlocked, behind your head. Exhale and raise your back up, bringing your left elbow towards the right knee, crunching the abdomen. Inhale and return to the start position. Repeat on the other side. Perform required number of repetitions.

Reverse Crunch

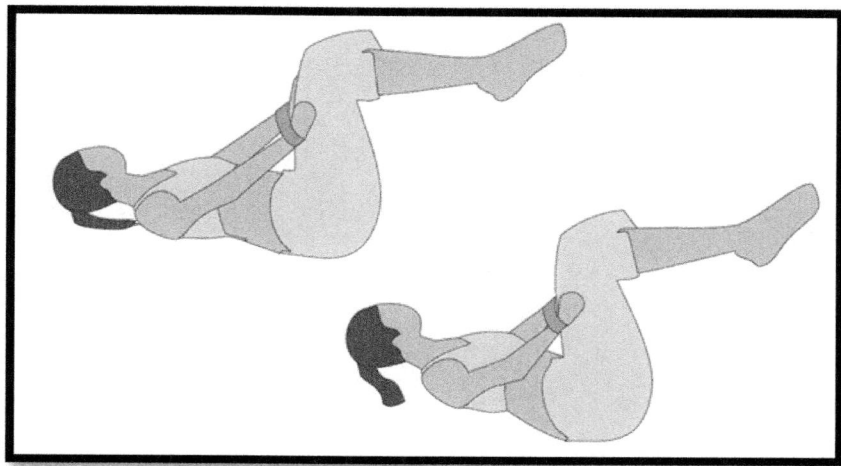

Lie down on your back with your legs bent at 90 degrees at hip and knees. Hold the resistance band in down grip against the lower part of thigh, just above the knees with your arms by side of your body. Imprint your back contracting your abdominals, roll your hips up, taking your knees towards the face as you raise your upper body slightly above the ground. With each crunch press your hands towards the feet, pushing against the resistance of the band. Try to keep your neck and shoulders relaxed and don't lock your elbows during the exercise. Perform required number of repetitions.

COOL-DOWN EXERCISES

Cool down exercises should always be performed after intensive workout to bring the body back to its normal state. Full body stretches are good cool down exercises. The body is in a very compliant state after exercises. Thus the stretches performed at this time help to increase the flexibility of the body.

Cool down stretch guidelines
1. Move into the stretched position (where you can feel slight tension) slowly.
2. Inhale and exhale deeply and slowly and let the stretching muscle relax.
3. Hold the stretch for 15 seconds and then slowly return to start position.
4. Perform each stretch twice.

Some stretches which are very beneficial for the body are as follows:

Upper Body Stretch

1. Triceps Stretch (Forward Arm Stretch):

Major muscles worked - rhomboids, deltoids and triceps brachii. Stand tall with your shoulders levelled and facing forwards and feet hip width distance apart. Extend your right arm to the side at shoulder level with palm facing forward. Move the arm forward and take it across the chest as if to wrap your chest with your arm.

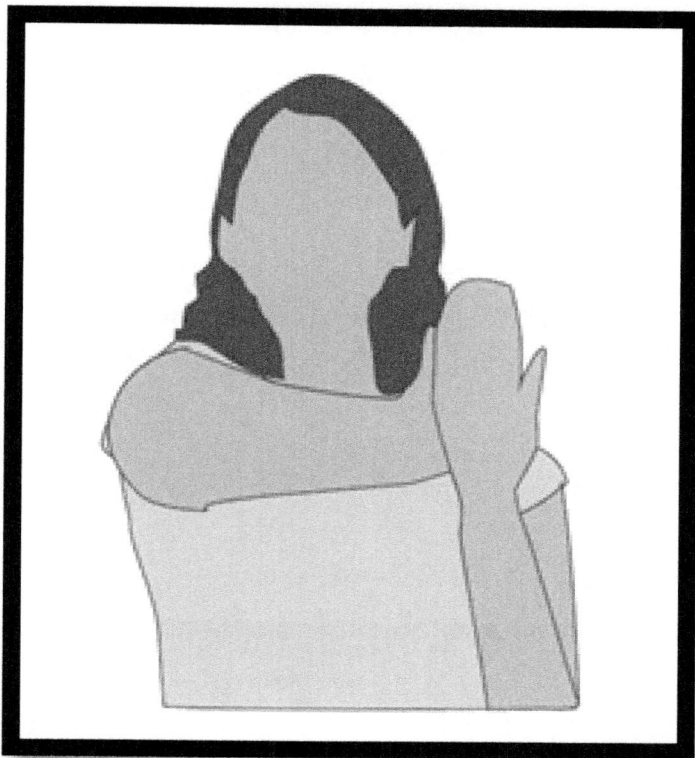

Bring the right hand around your left shoulder blade walking your fingertips towards your upper spine to the extent it is comfortable. Feel the stretch on the outside of your right arm, right shoulder and upper back. Breathe deeply into the thoracic spine and upper back, trying to release the stretching muscles. To increase the stretch you may give a slight push at the elbow of the wrapped arm, pulling it towards your chest. Relax. Repeat the above procedure for the left side.

2. <u>Pectoral Stretch (Backward Arm Stretch)</u>:

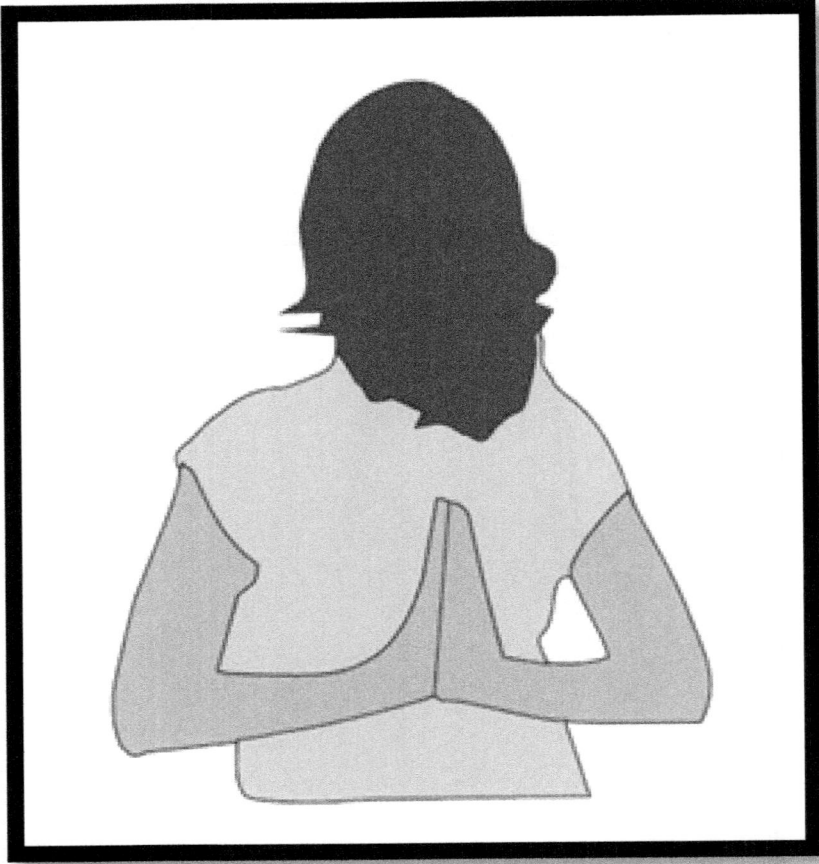

Major muscles worked - pectoralis major and deltoids. Stand tall with your shoulders levelled and facing forward and feet hip width distance apart. Extend your arms to the sides making a "T". Bend your arms at the elbows and bring both hands behind your back till the tip of middle fingers touch each other with little fingers of both hands pressing against the back. Start pushing the middle fingers up slowly. Try to bring all the fingers of left hand in contact with fingers of right hand. Slide the fingers up the spine till the stretch is comfortable. Inhale deeply while stretching the muscles of shoulder, chest, arms and fingers, relaxing them.

3. <u>Latissimus Dorsi And Triceps Stretch (Upward Arm Stretch)</u>:

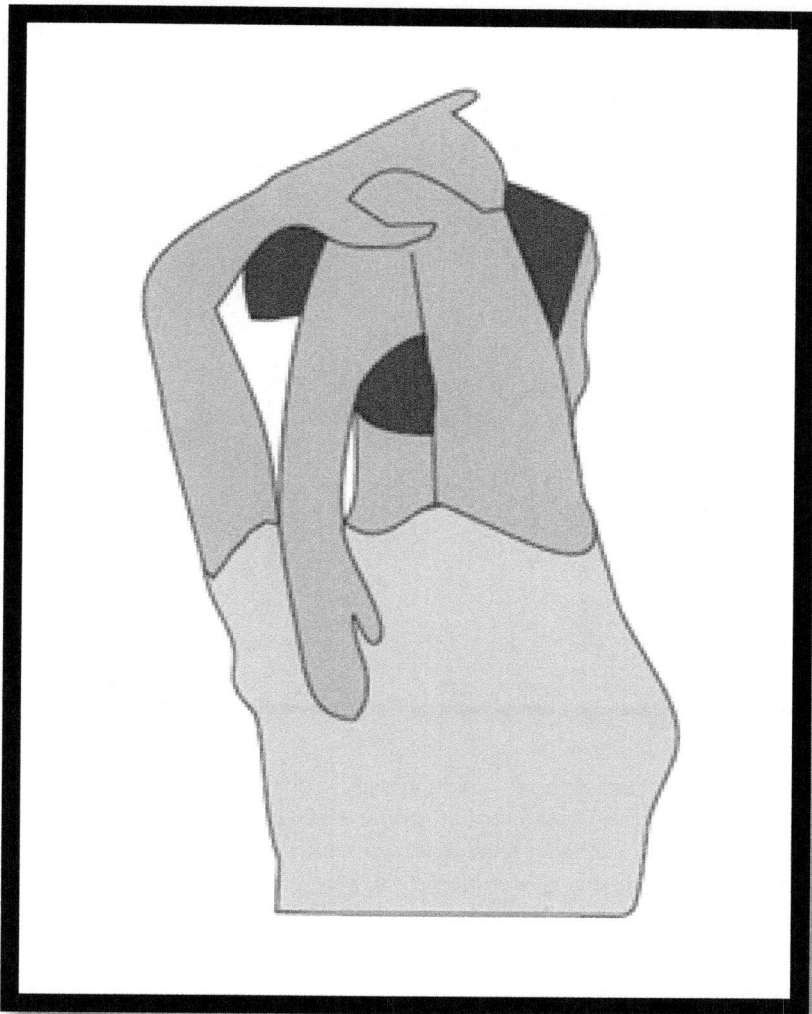

Major muscles worked - Latissimus dorsi and Triceps brachii
Extend your right arm to the side with palm facing up. Raise the arm
towards the ceiling and then bend at the elbow till your fingertips reach the
spine between your shoulder blades. Walk your fingertips down the spine.
Feel the stretch on the outer side of your right arm, upper back and the
right side of your trunk. Hold this position and breathe deeply trying to
release the stretching muscles of the upper back and around the spine.
Come to the start position. Repeat the above procedure for the left side.

Lower Body Stretch

1. <u>Figure Of Four Forward Bend:</u>

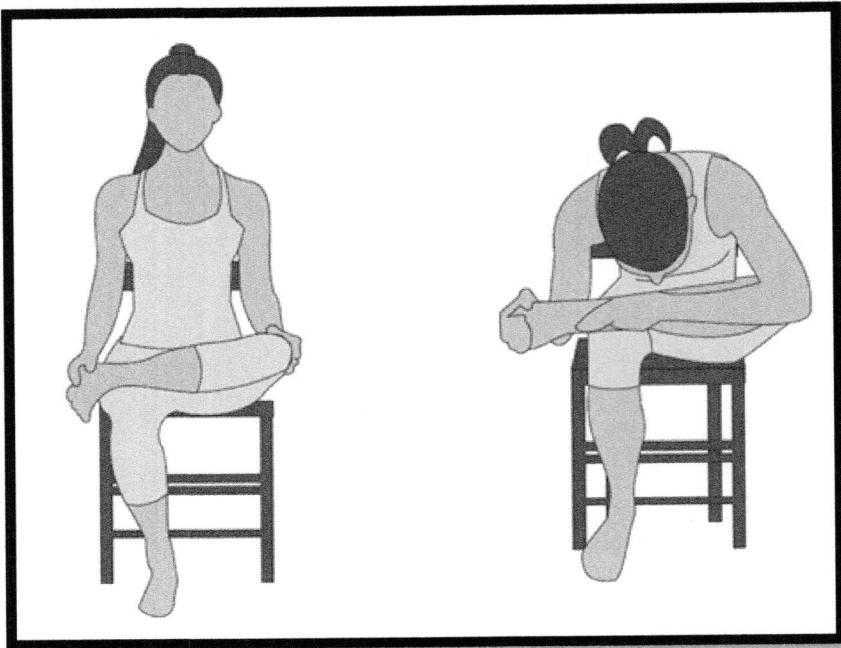

Major muscles worked - gluteus maximus and erector spinae.
Sit tall with feet firmly placed on the ground, hip width distance apart. Place your left ankle over the right knee making a figure of 4 with the legs. Stretch your spine in this position trying to free your hip joint. Let the knee go down under the effect of gravity, opening the left hip joint. Bend forward from this position, leading with your chest while still looking ahead. Breathe while stretching and release the spine and hip joint slowly. Drop your body down towards the floor. Feel the increase in stretch in the hip and spine region. Hold this position. To come out of the above position, raise your spine up, keeping it straight while still keeping the neck and shoulders relaxed. Keep pushing through the right foot into the ground to maintain balance. As the spine comes in an upright position, raise the head and look in front. Come to the start position. Repeat on the other side.

2. Thigh Stretch (Quadriceps Stretch):

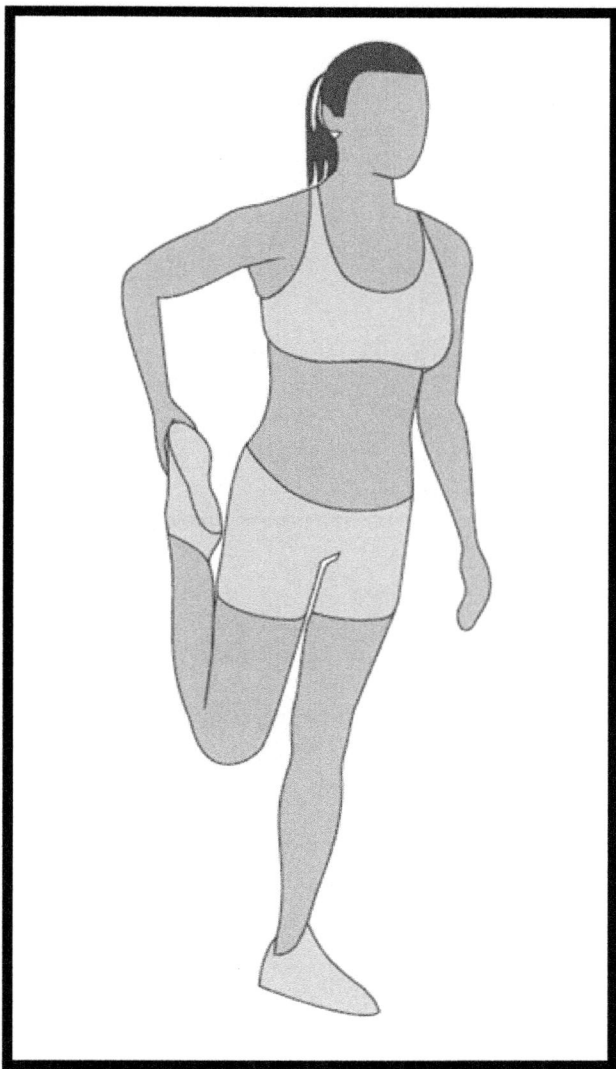

Stand tall with your abdomen tucked in and feet hip width distance apart.
Hold a wall or stationary object for balance, Grasp your left foot with your
left hand and pull so that your left heel moves towards your left buttock
(maintain proper alignment to avoid stress on your knee). You should feel
the stretch along the front of your left thigh. Repeat on the other leg.

3. Hamstring Stretch:

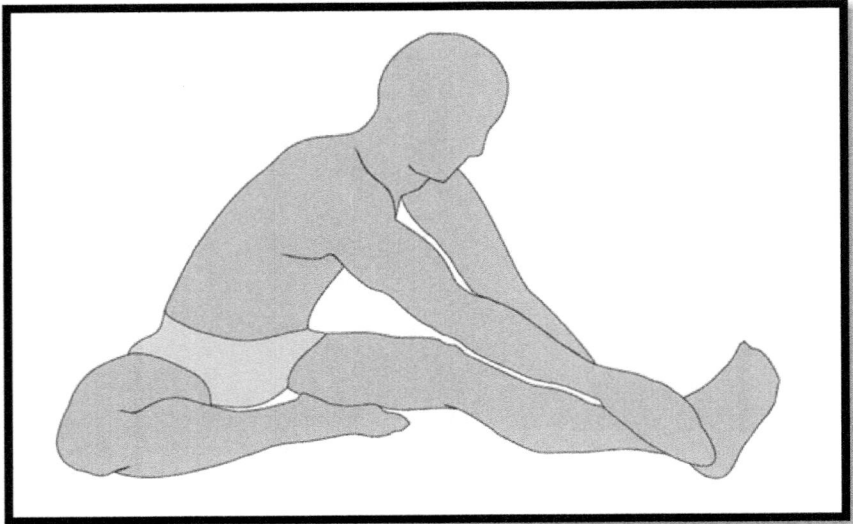

Major muscles worked - Hamstrings and erector spinae. Sit tall in a long sitting position on the floor with your legs hip width distance apart and stretched in front of you. Bend your right leg and place the sole of right foot against the inner side of left thigh, above the knee. Keep your shoulders and hips squared (facing forward). Bend forward at your hips (keeping your back straight and leading with the heart) and move your torso towards your left knee. Be sure to keep your left leg in neutral position with your left toes pointing up. Feel the stretch in your back and hamstring muscles. Switch the leg and repeat on the other side keeping your right leg stretched in front of you.

4. Calf Muscle Stretch:

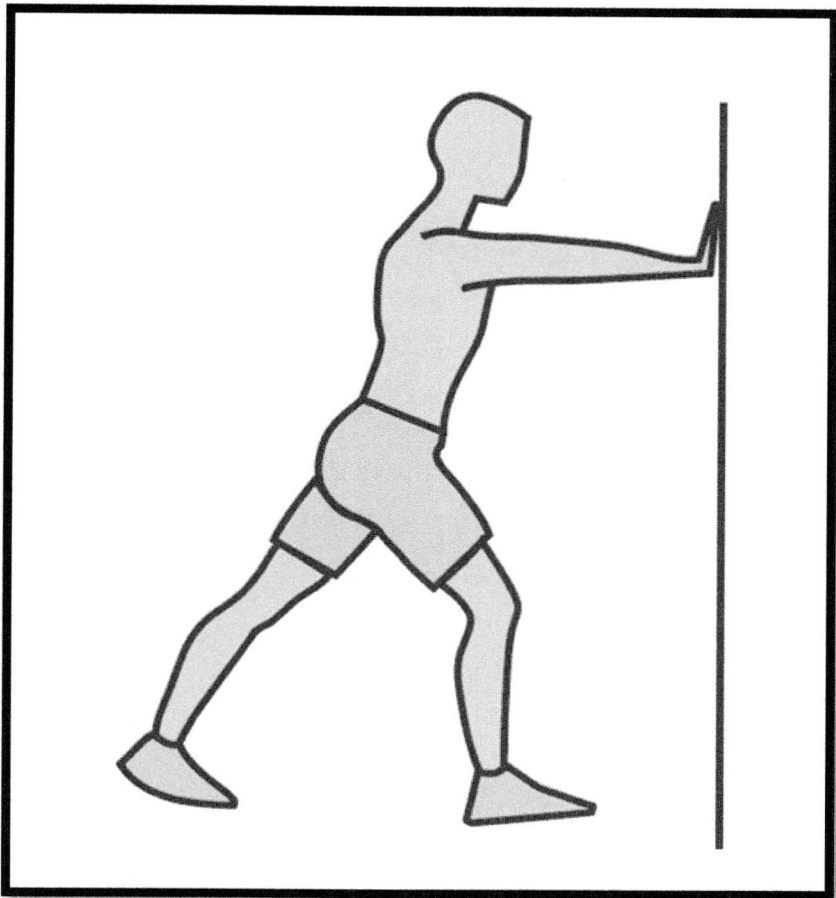

Major muscles involved: Soleus and gastrocnemius.

Stand with your right foot flat on the floor about 1 foot away from the wall (right leg bent) and the left leg stretched straight behind with left heel touching the floor. Place your hands on the wall and bend forwards, keeping your back straight. Feel the stretch behind your left leg. Repeat on the other side.

TRAINING REGIMES

BEGINNERS PROGRAM (ONE CIRCUIT)

MONDAY	UPPER BODY WORKOUT	Biceps Curls (15 rep.)
		Horizontal Arm Extensions (15 rep.)
		Rear Arm Extensions (15 rep.)
		Hand Scrunches (15 rep.)
		Vertical Arm Extensions (15 rep.)
	ABDOMINAL REGION WORKOUT	Abdominal Crunches (15 rep.)
		Bicycles (15 rep.)
		Reverse Crunches (15 rep.)
	LOWER BODY WORKOUT	Slide Clamshell (15 rep.)
		Standing Hip Adductions (15 rep.)
		Leg Extensions (15 rep.)
		Bridge Thrusts (15 rep.)

		Internal Rotations
		External Rotations
TUESDAY	Rest	
WEDNESDAY	UPPER BODY WORKOUT	Triceps Extensions (15 rep.)
		Vertical Arm Extensions (15 rep.)
		Lateral Pulldown (15 rep.)
		Bear Crawls (10 rep.)
		Seated Concentration Curls (15 rep.)
	ABDOMINAL REGION WORKOUT	Abdominal Crunch (15 rep.)
		Reverse Crunch (15 rep.)
		Oblique Overhead Extensions (15 rep.)
	LOWER BODY WORKOUT	Thigh Thrusts (15 rep.)
		Bridge Thrusts (10 rep.)
		Standing Hip Abductions (15 rep.)
		Single Leg Loop Bridge
		Internal Rotations
		External Rotations
THURSDAY	Rest	
FRIDAY	UPPER BODY WORKOUT	Horizontal arm extension (15 rep.)
		Triceps extension (15 rep.)
		Wrist curls (15 rep.)

		Hand crunch (15 rep.)
		Vertical arm extension (15 rep.)
	ABDOMINAL REGION WORKOUT	Abdominal crunch (15 rep.)
		Bicycles (15 rep.)
		Reverse crunch (15 rep.)
	LOWER BODY WORKOUT	Hip adduction (15 rep.)
		Bridge thrust (10 rep.)
		Band squats (10 rep.)
		Sitting leg raise (15 rep.)
		Internal rotation
		External rotation

WEEK WISE CIRCUIT ROUTINE

WEEK 1	Complete 1 circuit
WEEK 2	Complete 2 circuits with 2 minutes' gap between them
WEEK 3	Complete 3 circuits with 2 minutes' gap between 2 circuits
WEEK 4	Complete 4 circuits with 2 minutes' gap between 2 circuits

INTERMEDIATE PROGRAM

MONDAY	Repeat 4 circuits of beginners' Monday regime with the resistance one level higher than the one used in week 4. Increase the repetitions of Abdominal Crunches, Bicycles, Reverse Crunches & Bridge Thrusts to 15*2 repetitions per circuit.
TUESDAY	Rest
WEDNESDAY	Repeat 4 circuits of beginners' Wednesday exercise regime with the resistance one level higher than the one used in week 4. Increase the repetitions of Abdominal Crunches, Reverse Crunches, Oblique Overhead Extensions and Bridge Thrusts to 15*2 repetitions per circuit.
THURSDAY	Rest
FRIDAY	Repeat 4 circuits of beginners' Friday exercise regime with the resistance one level higher than the one used in week 4. Increase the repetitions of Hand Scrunches, Abdominal Crunches, Bicycles, Reverse Crunches and Bridge Thrusts to 20*2 repetitions per circuit.

Repeat intermediate regime for 4 weeks. Increase the resistance level of the band, when you are comfortable with one resistance level.

ADVANCED TRAINING (SPLIT TRAINING)

MONDAY	Repeat 4 circuits of beginners' Monday upper body regime with maximum resistance loop band. Oblique Overhead Extensions (25 rep.) Abdominal Crunches with Rotation (25 rep.)
TUESDAY	Repeat 4 circuits of beginners' Monday lower body regime with maximum resistance loop band. Bicycles (25 rep.) Reverse Crunches (25 rep.)
WEDNESDAY	Rest
THURSDAY	Repeat 4 circuits of beginners' Wednesday upper body regime with maximum resistance loop band. Oblique Overhead Extensions (25 rep.) Abdominal Crunches with Rotation (25 rep.)
FRIDAY	Repeat 4 circuits of beginners' Wednesday lower body regime with maximum resistance loop band. Bicycles (25 rep.) Reverse Crunches (25 rep.)

BONUS

We hope you liked the book and have already started doing these exercises.

You can get more tips & motivation to do these exercises by joining our mailing list. This would also ensure that an new learnings that I have related to this area are shared with you first. To join my mailing list, simply go to

http://www.fitness-sutra.com/erlb

ABOUT THE AUTHOR

Dr. Monika Chopra is a senior Physiotherapist and Therapeutic Yoga teacher with diverse experience and interests. She is working in the field of physiotherapy for past 13 years. She understands injuries and pain very closely.

Dr. Monika is registered with Indian Association of Physiotherapists. She specializes in the field of Orthopaedic, Neuromuscular physiotherapy and lifestyle related health problems. She is attached with reputed hospitals in Pune. She works as freelance ergonomic consultant to various well known organizations and companies. She also conducts seminars on postural corrections and office ergonomics. She arranges employee wellness workshops in various corporate sectors for orthopaedic rehabilitation and postural care.

Printed in Great
Britain
by Amazon